PRAISE FOR *LIKE WATER IS FOR FISH*

'It has been a real privilege to be associated with this book. Especially because very few people see the need to honour and celebrate stories. Many will tell you they do not have a story to tell. But without stories it would be like travelling naked through life. Indeed, we need our stories like fish need water. Thank you, Garth, for this reawakening. We will happily travel with you to the magic story island.'
– GCINA MHLOPHE

'Garth Japhet has a story worth listening to – as we all do.'
– ZAPIRO

'Garth Japhet believes in the power of story to change the world. His story shows you why, and invites us all to join his vision of a society transformed and living out its values. This book will inspire you to be a part of making this dream a reality. Highly recommended.'
– GRAEME CODRINGTON

'This beautifully and sensitively written book, exhibiting marvellous powers of description, will help you discover the power and significance of your own story and show you how to help others find theirs.'
– MICHAEL CASSIDY

'This book is Garth Japhet's invitation to dismantle some of your assumptions and to set down burdens of prejudice because his story looks

more like yours and mine than you realise, and that's the point really.'
– UFRIEDA HO

'This is a beautiful, powerful book. It showed me how little I really know a friend I thought I knew. From now on, no more assumptions or judgements, just grace and understanding towards every person who crosses my path.'
– MICHAEL MOL

'This book is a powerful, poignant and ultimately humble call to courage – courage to ask and then to listen to the stories of those around us. With a golden thread of empathy, Garth weaves vulnerable and brave storytelling together with a challenge to each one of us to harness the incredible power of story to affect change in our own lives and in the lives of those around us.'
– DEBORAH KIRSTEN

LIKE WATER IS FOR FISH

'Story is for a human as water is for a fish – all encompassing and not quite palpable.'
– JONATHAN GOTTSCHALL, author of *The Storytelling Animal: How Stories Make Us Human*

LIKE WATER IS FOR FISH

THE POWER OF STORY IN OUR LIVES

GARTH JAPHET

MACMILLAN

First published in 2021
by Pan Macmillan South Africa
Private Bag X19
Northlands
Johannesburg
2116
South Africa

www.panmacmillan.co.za

ISBN 978-1-77010-644-4
E-ISBN 978-1-77010-645-1

Editing by Alison Lowry
Proofreading by Sally Hines
Design and typesetting by Nyx Design
Cover design by publicide

MIX
Paper from
responsible sources
FSC   FSC® C022948
www.fsc.org

Printed by **novus print**, a division of Novus Holdings

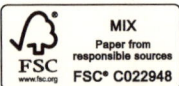

To my wife Jayne – my love story.

To my children Rebecca and Leigh – whose stories are just beginning …

To my dad – I wish I had asked you for your story while I had a chance.

To my mum – I'm glad I got to hear your story.

To my siblings Dee, Miles and Xan, whose lives and families are part of my story.

To my Soul City, Heartlines and forgood colleagues, without whom there wouldn't be much of a story to tell.

To all the people I have interviewed – thank you for sharing your stories with me.

To Alison – the unsung hero of this story, without whose encouragement and writing brilliance this story would never have seen the light of day.

To the Author of my story.

CONTENTS

INTRODUCTION

The epigraph which you may have noticed at the beginning of this book is worth repeating here:

> 'Story is for a human as water is for a fish – all encompassing and not quite palpable.'

They are the words of academic Jonathan Gottschall, whose book *The Storytelling Animal* is a fascinating blend of science and the humanities, demonstrating how story in its multiple and many-faceted forms affects our lives without us even noticing it. In an interview with Maria Konnikova of *Scientific American* in 2012, Gottschall said: '... the idea for this specific book came to me not from research but from a song. I was driving down the highway and happened to hear the country music artist Chuck Wicks singing "Stealing Cinderella" – a song about a little girl growing up to leave her father behind. Before I knew it, I was blind from tears, and I had to veer off on the road to get control of myself and to mourn the time – still more than a decade off – when my own little girls would fly the nest. I sat there on the side of the road feeling sheepish and wondering, "What just happened?"'

In putting this book together, the 'What just happened?' but also the 'What now?' have resonated continuously in my head.

In a 2am epiphany, I was struck by how stories, like some kind of hidden power, had shaped my choices, beliefs and sense of purpose. As a young boy the Jungle Doctor series of books had so captured me that against all advice and despite neither scientific interest nor aptitude, I

1

had set my heart on becoming a doctor. Then as a doctor who was more interested in health than in disease, I stumbled upon the healing power of story – fictional, factual and my own. Having been inspired by story, I had begun to tell stories to inspire. What magic was at work here?

It was this question that set me on the journey that would become this book. It is my hope that as you accompany me on this journey, you will become more aware of this hidden power that permeates and influences every aspect of our lives.

This book is not an autobiography; nor is it a memoir in the conventional sense. Rather I have chosen to tell stories from my own life that illustrate how story has influenced me and how I have used it to influence others. It has also been my privilege to interview a wide range of amazing people, specifically for this project and to hear from them the impact of story on their lives. (Strangely, it was easier to ask for an interview to talk about story than to raise funding …) Some are well known for their high profile as performers, business people, speakers who make their living on stages or by strategic thinking and consultation in a broad variety of arenas. Some of their names may be familiar, others not. There are singers, artists, academics and activists. Many are associates of mine, colleagues or friends, while others are people I met for the first time. All of these people have one thing in common – the recognition of what we all know instinctively, namely, the transformative power of story. And all of them have something that is unique to them: they have their individual stories to own and to share. They have done so generously here.

As I began to write, I discovered that the book had its own ideas, which it would reveal to me in its own good time. But like a good thriller, the unveiling happened in fits and starts and was littered with heartbreaking dead ends and unexpected revelations. Finally, it coalesced into the four distinct but overlapping themes that make up the book.

Each section sets out to explore a core theme but the stories, anecdotes and life-turning moments or events often interweave, one with another. Such as how understanding our own story helps us and others. How being curious about the stories of others is a simple way to bring healing and empathy to a fractured world. And how story is the most effective way to persuade and influence people, whether to change behaviour, sell a product or lead a team. There is also a smattering of neuroscience showing how science has proved what humanity intuitively already knew, namely, that our brains are wired for story.

The themes are illustrated by parts of my own narrative and, at the end of each section under the sub-heading 'In Others' Words', by the voices of those people I interviewed.

The thematic structure is deliberate, the underlying intention being to demonstrate a progression, and the book is divided into four parts. Part 1: Shaping – The Gift of Knowing Your Own Story speaks to the importance of understanding our foundations, the things and people who shape and impact our lives at foundational moments. Part 2: Framing – The Riches of Imagination, the Poverty of Assumption explores the multiple ways in which stories may be framed, constructed, recounted and received. It pulls into focus the assumptions we make about others, how quick we are to judge and devalue, and how much the poorer we are for moving to hasty conclusions before taking the time to listen and try to understand. Part 3: Believing – Holding the Faith is about dreams imagined, shattered, rebuilt or reconfigured. It is about keeping a vision alive when hard evidence paints a dismal picture or when mentally and spiritually the terrain ahead appears impenetrable. It speaks to issues of mental health and the ongoing struggles many people, myself included, have to navigate – in dealing with stigma, and the impact of talking openly and sharing a journey that, at times, can feel dark and very lonely. Part 4: Influencing – The Power of Story to Challenge Thinking and Change Behaviour is a demonstration of the way story may be used to influence others in positive and powerful ways.

Because of this loosely containing structure, my personal story does not always flow chronologically, but it is the thread that holds the pattern to its course, looping backwards and forwards in the way my life has unfolded, and continues to unfold, and the many challenges and dark nights of the soul, as well as the joys, I have experienced along the way.

I hope that as you read this book you will be surprised by the power of story and recognise how central it is to our human experience. That you will be encouraged to engage with story in all its many facets; to understand yourself and others, to inspire, to influence and even to heal.

PART 1

SHAPING – THE GIFT OF KNOWING YOUR OWN STORY

In my mid-20s, at a time when I was trying to make sense of what seemed to me like a life in a mess, I was encouraged and supported to review my life story. At first I was sceptical. It seemed very self-indulgent, very navel-gazing. What good could it do to review a past that couldn't be changed? I saw it as an exercise in futility. How wrong I was.

Despite my misgivings, I agreed to try. I was guided to identify and revisit specific periods and events in my life, from my childhood through to the present, and see them through a new, more positive lens.

I came to realise what perhaps should be a simple, obvious truth. It is important first to go within, to look deeply into the things that shape us, to understand context and nuance, to acknowledge those who were present – and absent – during our formative years and the roles they played in how we behave and how we came to view the world. Accepting and owning your personal story is an invaluable gift.

For me, the process enabled me to understand myself better – and often forgive myself. It also allowed me to deepen relationships by helping others understand me better.

I came to realise that my story has not only been shaped by my relationships and lineage but that it is inexorably intertwined with the story of my country and its people. Understanding my country's story and recognising and acknowledging how differently it has impacted on my life and the lives of others has been an equally enriching experience.

But the greatest gift in knowing my story has been the opportunity to share it and so potentially bring understanding, inspiration and sometimes healing to others.

In researching material for this book, I found that reams have been written about the power of reviewing your personal story. Studies have been done to show the amazing power that reframing our narratives can have on our lives. There is even a whole field of clinical practice, Narrative Psychology, which positions helping people 'rewrite' their stories at the core of their healing work. How what seems like a disaster can turn out to have been a turning point in the journey, as Jonathan Sacks explores in his book *Morality: Restoring the Common Good in Divided Times*, the final destination of which is more remarkable than might have been otherwise.

In Part 1, I describe some of my journey of exploration into my personal story. In the section at the end, 'In Others' Words', is the testimony of some of the many people I interviewed during my research, who shared their individual understanding of the gift of story with me.

1.

SOME CHILDREN

At the age of five, I was officially a nursery school dropout. I lasted one, single day – and when my mother said I did not have to go back for another, it felt like a victory.

It meant I could stay at home with Mum and have her all to myself, while my much older siblings were at school and my father at work.

I knew I did not have any friends my own age, but that was okay. I did not need new friends. I did not need to learn how to play with others. I did not need to navigate a terrifying world full of chaos and colours and children running and shouting and shoving.

I had my books – and I had my mother, who read me stories.

I had Serena, who looked after me with care and devotion as if I was her own child. Her smile was as wide as the world and her soft, strong hands smelled of Lifebuoy soap and Vaseline. Safe hands. I knew those hands better than my mother's. They washed and fed me, comforted and scolded me.

And I had Ben, tall as a giraffe, my companion and daytime confidante, who would occasionally let me ride with him on his bicycle to visit his friends or, for a treat, conjure up a steaming yellow enamel mug of 'Bennie's Special Tea' with spoonfuls of sugar in it. On tea days, I would sit on an upended paint tin, complete with cardboard cushion, outside his room behind our house. We would slurp our tea and munch our slabs of white bread in contented silence.

Serena Mojapelo and Ben Sibanda. I knew almost nothing about them or about their lives. All I knew was that I missed them terribly when, once a year, they went on holiday.

I couldn't wait for them to come home.

I REMEMBER MY first day of school as if it were yesterday.

Serena bustles into my room, her red apron swishing against her legs.

'Wake up, my boy. It's a big day, Garthy! You must be so excited for your first day at school.'

The whiteness of her headscarf contrasts against the smooth dark skin of her smiling face.

I look up at her. 'Yes,' I say, but I think I mean no.

'Let's get you up and dressed then, so you won't be late.'

She moves to the window and I watch her draw back the curtains, letting in a cascade of morning light, casting zebra shadows over me, which disappear as soon as Serena frees me from my cot.

At five I still sleep in a bed with cot-sides.

'Serena, my tummy is sore, I don't feel well,' I say as she sets me on the floor.

'Garthy, I am making you your favourite breakfast, bacon and eggs. You will need your strength for school.'

School. The sick feeling in my stomach gets worse.

'What happens if I am sick at school and they can't find Mummy?'

My imagination fires viscously, transporting me into the strange environment I imagine school to be. No Serena, no Mum, just lots of children and adults I don't know. Adrenalin courses through my body, whacking first into my heart, beating it out of my chest, then colliding with my brain, sending my thoughts spinning.

Serena senses my panic. She dresses me gently. 'You will be fine, Garthy, you are a big boy now. Think of all those friends you can play with.'

I am unconvinced.

I ALWAYS HEAR Mum before I see her. Step, thump, step. Her gammy leg drags over the floorboards.

She stands in the doorway of the kitchen, where I am sitting at the table moving my congealing breakfast around my plate.

'Time to go, darling,' she says.

'I don't feel well, Mummy, my tummy is sore,' I say.

She is pale, but goes paler. 'Come on, darling, don't make a fuss. It's just a little bit of nerves, butterflies in the stomach.' Her anxiety cascades off her and wafts over me like a strong perfume.

We make it to the car. Our car looks like a penguin, black and white with rear swooping wings. Inside the seats are of red leather. My sweaty palms leave a mottled shadow on the gleaming chrome door handle. The wind soon restores the handle to its brilliance, but when we have reached our destination, as I climb out and close the door behind me the shadow returns, denser this time.

It's a blur. Children, lots of them, shouting, laughing, running. An avalanche of noise and colour. I shrink back against Mum's leg, holding tight.

A woman wearing a beige cardigan stretched over her generous front, the sort of front that can envelop and comfort, comes towards us. 'You must be Garth,' she says.

'Yes,' I stammer.

'I'm Sheila, your teacher,' she says. 'Now let's get you settled. Come and meet some of the children in your class.' She is down on her haunches, smiling, looking me in the eye, holding out her hand. She looks how grannies should look. The tortoise-shell comb possibly intended to tame her wild tangle of greying brown hair is half falling out. She smells as grannies should, of butterscotch sweets.

But she is not Mum and she is not Serena and I am scared. It feels as though I am going into a dark tunnel away from the light, and every instinct, every nerve ending is screaming Flee! I start to cry. To wail. 'Nooo, Mummy, don't leave me ...' I cling to my mother's leg like a limpet. She tries to wrench herself away and turns her head, but not before I can see the tears in her eyes.

Somehow Sheila, looking heavenward, manages to pry me away from Mum, who limps back to the car.

My wailing has momentarily stopped some of the children at play and they look at me curiously. Then a bell clangs and they all start running. Sheila holds my hand tightly and I am pulled, still crying, towards the classroom.

This is not a quiet place, not like my home where the loudest noises are the swoosh, splash, swoosh of Serena's mop progressing down the passage and the whisper of my book's pages turning. This is loud and chaotic and frightening.

I am led towards a desk with two wooden chairs, blue book bags hanging off their backs.

'Come now, Garth, you sit here next to Simon. There, there. You'll soon feel better.'

Simon, a small, freckled boy, not unlike myself, looks up. 'Hi,' he says.

'Hi,' I say back, hiccuping.

I don't remember much else of that morning, just a confused series of events and images punctuated by milk, sandwiches and play time. I stay at my desk. No one is nasty to me; some boys even ask me to play. I just don't know how to play. Will Mum remember to fetch me?

My tears dry in the course of the morning and when I am not thinking about home, I think I like it here. That is, until the next morning, when it's time to come back.

'WAKEY, WAKEY,' SERENA says, as she moves to open the curtains.

'Wakey, wakey' assumes that I am sleeping. I am not. My eyes are open and wild, and my mind is grappling with a torrent of images.

Me, left at school. Me, sick. Me, abandoned.

It is crazy stuff but it is also very real. I cling with desperation onto the cot-sides as Serena comes to pick me up. 'Nooo,' I wail. 'I don't want to go back to schoool …'

'But you must, Garthy, you are a big boy now.'

'Nooo ...' I cling harder.

Serena sighs.

Mum gives in almost immediately. I think she is actually relieved at my refusal.

And so a pattern is set.

FIRST THERE IS primary school, Grade 1 at The Ridge. Same script – although this time I up my game and I manage a week.

My sisters are at Roedean, which is mostly an all-girls school, but it does accept a few boys (three, among 500 or so girls – I did not know how lucky I was). So off I go to Roedean and because my sisters are there, it feels safe. I complete Grade 1 and Grade 2 and I am happy.

Then it's back to The Ridge. Mrs Locke, my Grade 2 teacher, is beautiful. At seven years old I think I love her. Yes, Grade 2 again; I have been kept back a year. This is not because I am not okay academically, but rather the parent/teacher wisdom believing that being older in the class should help me. They are right. It does help.

I still get anxious; my imagination still insists that I will get sick at school and they won't be able to find Mum. But I've worked this out. If I really, really worry about something – like a test, a school outing, or being left at school – then whatever it is that I fear won't happen. But if I *don't* worry, then ... So I have a licence to worry and I do.

The Ridge is a high-water mark. Seven full years and no dropping out. I make friends. I become famous for what's under my fingernails when I grow a world-beating, multi-coloured forest of fungi in a petri dish. (Forty-five years later, people are still talking about it.)

I make my theatrical debut in a series of ghoulish roles, first as the wizard in the *Wizard of Oz*, closely followed by my starring role as the First Witch in *Macbeth* (they didn't have to use much make-up). In athletics, I win the 200 metres using a cunning plan: stroll the first 100, let the others tire themselves out and then go like a bat out of hell in the last 100. It works! Inadvertently, I learn how to develop photographs when, for the last six months of school, I am consigned to the darkroom by my French teacher.

THWACK! THE SQUASH ball hurtles towards me. I reflexively duck, spin and scoop it off the back wall. My return shot grazes the court side, making Craig run. He stretches, and with a flick of his wrist he drops the ball over the tin and into the corner. Game set and match. He smiles good-naturedly, sweat dripping from the end of his nose.

'That was so close.'

'Yes, close but not close enough!' I retort. 'You always beat me.'

Craig and I have been friends since we were seven years old. If he'd been born in the United States he would have been that 'all American boy', sporty, good-looking, clever, popular. And me? Less the good-looking part – I am thirteen and acne and braces are not exactly attractive – but sporty, clever and popular: tick.

'You coming to prep now?'

'No, I'm seeing Mr Rodgers.'

'Trouble?'

'No, nothing serious.'

But it is serious.

For weeks I have been feeling as though I am falling, while standing on solid ground. My terror-laden thoughts have been scrambling for purchase and it's getting worse. It's completely irrational. I know that.

I am in my first term at Michaelhouse, a boarding school in the KwaZulu-Natal Midlands. The school, an assortment of turreted red brick and stone buildings, is tucked up against the foot of the undulating foothills of the Drakensberg. Beautifully manicured playing fields are bordered by avenues of oak trees, home to squadrons of cicadas that screech endlessly on a hot summer day. At least I think that's their home but I have never seen them. At night frogs in the nearby stream (which, inexplicably, is called 'the bog stream') compete with the daytime cicadas. I prefer the frogs – they're more melodic.

I love it here and yet the feeling of desperation and impending doom just grows and grows.

Later that afternoon I sit in a high-backed, leather-upholstered chair facing my tweed-clad housemaster.

'Explain to me why you are unhappy,' Mr Rodgers says. 'Are you being bullied?'

'No,' I sob, snot and tears dribbling off my chin, and it's true – I'm not being bullied. 'I don't know why, but I just want to go home.'

It's been the same pattern for the last few weeks. Poor Mr Rodgers. I can see that he is desperately trying to help, but it's hard to fix something when nothing is wrong.

'Perhaps you're sick? Let's ask Matron to have a look at you.'

I am less than keen. I have been to see Matron already. She is, as you would expect a boys' school matron to be, an intimidating, no-nonsense woman, with hairs growing out of the moles on her chin. 'Give me your arm!' she had barked before plunging a needle into my vein. I presume it was a vein, but it might have been an artery because when I came to from my dead faint there was blood everywhere. I was not going back there in a hurry.

Until term ends I lead this strange double life. When I am busy I'm fine – in the choir, playing rugby and squash, and getting big-time street cred by winning the general knowledge event for my house ('What is the unit of measurement for food?' 'Kilojoules!'). But when I am not busy the pit returns. I wake up in the early hours of every morning, desperate. I am often on my knees in the chapel. 'God, please help me.'

When the end of term finally comes, I know that I can't go back. I will refuse to go back.

And when Mum says I am not going back to Michaelhouse, I am not going back.

DAY ONE AS a weekly boarder at St Alban's and the groundless terror is back. I can't explain it to anyone, not even to myself. I wade through the torture of the week with thoughts of home consuming my waking hours.

The weekend comes and I am not going back – again. Again Mum says, 'Okay, we will find another school for you.'

But this time I see the profound disappointment on Dad's face. He does not say anything, but I can see that I have let him down. For a young boy, to let your dad down is the worst feeling in the world.

I am not good enough, I am not man enough.

I look in the mirror and a gawky, spotty boy stares back. *You bloody failure. It's only the middle of the year and you have already been through two schools.* While I am feeling wretched, I don't think I am that surprised. I am, after all, the kid who dropped out of nursery school, lasted a week in Grade 1, went to an all-girls school for two years, got held back a year, couldn't crack Michaelhouse, and couldn't stick with St Alban's.

Now the only school that will take me is an inner-city school, a cram college, a last-resort place for kids who don't fit, kids with a drug habit. Maybe I would feel better about myself if I was on drugs.

I am not on drugs. I stick it out for six months before going back to a 'normal' school, St David's, where, in spite of my lack of scientific aptitude, I do well enough to get into medical school.

2.

GEORGE AND OTHER FRIENDS

'Dad, I have decided I want to become a doctor.'

My father looks up from his paper, confused. 'You what?'

I bulldoze on. 'Dad, I really want to be a doctor.'

He folds the paper, sighs. 'Where did this come from? You've never shown any aptitude or interest in maths or science and you are not even doing biology for matric!'

I feel a pang of sympathy for him. I have been a real headache over the last few years and now this.

'I don't know, Dad. I just know that that is what I want to be … I really want to make a difference to people's lives,' I say lamely.

My dad is a lawyer and he can spot faulty logic when he hears it. 'But you can do that by being a lawyer, as we agreed,' he points out. 'You're good at language, you debate well, why the change?'

I tell him about the Jungle Doctor – of which more later … My father is a kind man so he does not dismiss my thoughts.

'Okay, remember when I cut my hand you fainted at the sight of the blood?' I nod miserably. I know where this is headed. 'In fact, every time there's been a trace of blood you pass out. As a doctor you're going to have to swim in blood!'

He is right, of course. I could play to my strengths, become a lawyer, help people. But I can't tell him my real motives. Yes, it is about helping people, but as I am only to understand in later years, it is mainly about helping me.

I play the scripts out in my head.

'So, Lance, what's Garth doing next year?' 'Medicine,' is Dad's proud reply.

No, it doesn't feel that law holds the twin promises I crave: acceptance and desirability.

I set my heart on medicine.

And so, despite my C average for matric and A levels in English and history, which I do in England, for some reason known only to them, in 1981 I am accepted to do medicine at Wits.

THE POWER TO dream, to live out a story in your head, is one of humanity's greatest gifts. Without it we would be little different to the creatures around us. But a dream can also be like the trailer to a film; we get to see the most dramatic parts of the story, not the rest of it.

The story in my medical fantasy went something like this: failure boy confounds the naysayers to become a doctor, goes on radically to impact Africa, and wins fame, fortune and fair maid in the process. Rich in high points and short on minor details, such as how 'failure boy' gets to get his medical degree when this will involve studying pure sciences, for which he has little aptitude or passion.

This inconvenient question rears large in my mind as I stand, sweating, waiting to register for my first year of med school. The queue outside the administration building moves slowly. I look around. We are a fairly nondescript group of white men, with a smattering of white women, and even fewer students of either gender who would be classified 'Black', 'Coloured' and 'Indian'. If I'm honest, I am quite disappointed, everyone looks so normal. Not the 'cream of the cream' Professor Tobias had described us as at the welcome lecture.

'You are the chosen!' he had bellowed, and he should know. He is an expert on human evolution. A short greying man in his mid-50s with a disproportionally large head, he has been nominated three times for a Nobel Prize and is the Dean of Medicine at Wits. This group does not appear to be the pinnacle of human development. Not, that is, until I start talking to some of them. Their stories all seem intimidatingly similar. Violin virtuoso and Dux scholar, seven A's for matric (unheard of then), head boy, provincial water polo player, and, and, and … These were the type of matrics whose blazers seem to sag under the weight of their accolades. I feel completely out of place. How on earth am I going to get through this? Maybe I should have listened to Dad, and done law.

My musings are broken when the woman in front of me turns abruptly and, smiling enthusiastically, says, 'It's a miracle, isn't it?' I'm nonplussed.

'What is?' I stammer.

'That in six years we will be doctors able to do surgery, deliver babies. I find that mind-blowing.'

'Yes, it is,' I say. She has no idea what a miracle it would be in my case.

We introduce ourselves. Cheryl is slightly taller than me. She is wearing a flowing kaftan-type dress and leather sandals, and she radiates an infectious energy and enthusiasm. She's seriously nice, seriously bright and has the standard set of accolades – head girl, Dux scholar, etcetera. In a flash of inspiration I have a plan.

'Do you have a partner yet?' I ask her. She looks at me quizzically.

'Do I have a boyfriend?'

I blush. 'Uh, no … it's just that I've heard that for subjects like physics we need a partner and I wonder whether you would be mine?'

'Um, I …' I've caught her by surprise.

'You can always think about it,' I say quickly.

She hesitates and then smiles. 'Well, okay, why not?' she says.

And that is how I get through first year – and the years after that. Friends.

WHAT A PRIVILEGE it is to study the mysteries of the human body and what a blessing to do it with others. Few courses of study have the potential to forge such trust and depth of relationship. Medicine, like war, brings out the very best and worst in people; together you experience not only academic pressure but also the rawness of life, suffering, birth and death.

We make an interesting group. There is Johan, a bit of a mystic and older than the rest of us; flame-haired Erik, fresh from four years' theological training and soon to displace me as Cheryl's partner; tall, dipstick Mike with his vivid blue eyes; and dark-haired Tracy – friend to all us guys but, despite our best efforts, girlfriend to none. 'Ox-eye' Guy is a Brad Pitt look-alike from a banana farm on the South Coast, so named because in second year he ate (and chewed) a whole ox eye to win a bet. Fresh ox eyes were plentiful in second year: we were given them to dissect instead of the raisins that were the formalin-shrunken eyes of our cadavers.

Then there is Denis, who will become my partner though the clinical years and will save my butt on numerous occasions. We don't look that different, both of us have freckles, sandy brown hair and horrible gold-rimmed glasses. This alikeness, I believe, works in my favour as we are often confused, so much so that I'm convinced that I'm often awarded Denis's marks, which are usually better than mine. It will be Denis who catches the first baby I deliver when I am passed out cold.

Megan, short, blonde, fun and brighter than all of us, and not aware of it, is the love of Denis's life. He proposes to this amazing woman in fifth year and his bachelor party is a thing of legend. We get him thoroughly intoxicated, put both arms and legs in plaster, then leave him outside in wet clothes in mid-winter. Strangely, he becomes unresponsive. We try out our new medical skills to resuscitate him, give up and, finally, aware that he may need better care, get him admitted to our teaching hospital at 2am via a kindly matron. Fortunately, he recovers. At 5am we call Megan to pick him up. We ask her if she knows how to use a plaster saw. 'Why?' she asks. Needless to say, no one else dares to get married for the rest of our time at medical school.

The first three years are horrible. Incomprehensible subjects like biochemistry and biomaths, microanatomy and pharmacology, and then, just to confirm how ludicrous this all is, four hours of anatomy, picking bits off formalin-embalmed bodies every day for a whole year. You can tell a second-year student because they stink. If one of us had died that year, you could have left our body for weeks and still found it perfectly preserved.

Each morning my three ultra-studious dissection partners and I descend into the bowels of medical school to renew our relationship with 'George'. For me it is a descent into hell. We spend hours looking for minor structures like 'the lateral cutaneous nerve of the thigh', something so obscure that the knowledge of its existence might – *might* – be of use to a specialist surgeon. To get through the day, I find novel ways to break the monotony and the diligence of my partners, such as instructing them to link various pieces of anatomy with pieces of coloured wool to mark out 'important anatomical planes'.

Sometimes it is hours before they realise that George is the only body thus attired. But quite often, to their relief, I simply flee to the safety of the canteen and a good book.

As I write this, I wonder why I never thought of George as anything more than a scientific battle ground? What was George's story? What road had brought him to rest on that cold steel table? Perhaps there are some stories that are best left untold. I am not sure I could have picked him apart if he'd been human to me.

The clinical years prove to be better.

After three years of dreary lectures, dissection halls and laboratories, fourth year finally arrives and with it, the spectre of actually touching real patients. We cannot wait! We are like children who have been cooped up too long, desperate to get outside and play. Play for us is to examine, to use our shiny new stethoscopes, to stitch, to do whatever, as long as we are pressing flesh.

What a let-down. Our teachers admonish us if our hands so much as twitch. 'If I see one of you touch a patient before getting their story, there'll be hell to pay. That is the key to diagnosis. You only examine a patient to help you confirm what you already suspect.'

As much as it irked me then, I know now that this skill is at the very heart of healing. Long before the advent of modern medicine, listening to a patient's story was one of the few tools available to the physician. Science has since proved that the mere act of recounting their story to an empathetic listener helps people to cope with and even heal from their illness. It is especially helpful in dealing with loss or trying to make sense of their disease.

My disordered mind still struggles with the rigours of the meticulous and logical approach to diagnosis and treatment. I don't just have long dark nights of the soul. I have weeks and months of deep despair as I wrestle with the mismatch of my dreams, my aptitudes and my interests.

It is my group of amazing friends and my Jungle Doctor vision that help me through from one year to the next.

3.

MY COUNTRY HAS A STORY

The heat dances off the hard-packed red earth of the Voortrekkerhoogte parade ground. The air stagnates, moved only by the occasional barked command and shuffling of feet. I look around me at a thousand other young men, all of them, like me, freshly shorn. We are variegated shapes and sizes, but we have one thing in common: we are all white. And in the dying days of apartheid, the government is attempting to fashion us into soldiers.

'Japhet! Sak vir twintig, jou slegte ding!'

The corporal is a podgy boy whose moon-face has been severely assaulted by a combination of acne and the sun. I wouldn't be surprised if he was bullied at school and now that he has some power, he's going to use it. Funny how that works.

The reason I'm having to drop and do 20 press-ups is because I've questioned yet another inane parade ground instruction and now I must be punished.

'Ag, sorry, korporaal,' I say with mock sincerity, 'I can't do that.'

'Hoekom nie?' he shouts. He's not used to back chat.

'It will mess with my back,' I reply. 'I'm G3K3.'

He reddens even further, if that's possible, and scowls, but he knows there is nothing he can do. G3K3 means I'm medically fit enough to be in the army, but not to do press-ups.

'Ja, troep, you think you're clever with your degree, hey?' he sneers. 'Well, let me tell you, it means nothing in here. Nothing! You think you can get out of serving your country, but you can't!'

I stand my ground, but my insides have liquidised. There is only one law in here – their law.

'We're watching you, Japhet!'

I smile bravely, but after an uncomfortable second or two of waiting for what's coming, the corporal skulks off, scowling. Rivulets of sweat trace their way down my back and pool in the waistband of my shorts. I'm not sure whether it's the intensifying morning heat or fear.

One thing I am sure of is that this is a stuff-up. I've just started here and already these guys know my name. I've still got another four weeks of my basic training and if I don't get out of here soon my life will be hell. I don't think I'm brave enough for hell. How could I have been so dumb as to even think that my plan to arrive here only to be discharged immediately would work. I remonstrate with myself as I think back on the circumstances and the events that have brought me to this moment.

FOR ALL WHITE South African males, conscription was not negotiable. After you finished school, your call-up papers would arrive and that was that. It was possible to delay the fateful day with tertiary study, but sooner or later you would have to do your 'national duty'.

I had dragged out the fateful day, when I would need to decide to go or not go, but at the end of my medical internship I finally ran out of road. I needed to make a decision.

I understood people who felt they had to go into the army – but I couldn't. I grew up knowing, through my father in particular, that apartheid was wrong. I remember feeling a deep sense of injustice when black people were hauled off the street for not being able to produce their pass-books and, more often than not, thrown in jail. But it was only when I read Donald Woods' book *Biko* (banned in South Africa at the time) that I understood the true systematic and legislated horror of the system. Until then, I did not know Steve Biko's life story, nor the events that led up to him being killed by the police and the cover-up that followed. We were allowed only a part-version in apartheid South Africa in the 1970s, the version the authorities needed us to believe. When I read the real story I vowed, then and there, that I would never be part of the apartheid collusion and, if possible, I would fight against it.

One way of 'avoiding' conscription was to be a conscientious objector, but for me this wasn't an option. Conscientious objectors did not have an easy time of it and I knew that I didn't have the moral courage or mental strength required. The only other choice, one that I hated having to make but made nevertheless, was to leave the country. I made the decision to travel – with the UK as a first stop – and hoped that one day I could return and not have to serve a system I could not support in any shape or form.

After six months of oppressive skies and irregular locum jobs in the United Kingdom, I'd had enough. I looked farther afield. Very far, as it happened. I found a job as a medical officer in the town of Burnie in Tasmania. Burnie is a pin-prick on the backside of Tasmania, which in turn is a pin-prick on the backside of the world. Burnie! After being seduced through medical school with dreams of medical heroism and of being South Africa's own 'Jungle Doctor', I was going to Burnie!

However, at the end of 1989, just as I was about to leave for Australia, FW de Klerk threw me a lifeline (although maybe not personally) when he announced sweeping changes in South Africa. The unbanning of the ANC, release of political prisoners, including Nelson Mandela, and the beginning of 'talks' revealed the tantalising possibility of a new dawn in my home country.

I called the hospital in Burnie.

'So sorry, I'm afraid I need to turn down your job offer ...'

Silence. Then, 'Why?'

'I'm going back home. To do military service.'

'To do what?' my not-yet-boss asked incredulously.

I couldn't explain. I doubted his ability to understand my need to be part of a story bigger than myself, not as an observer but as an active participant, so I didn't even try.

All I knew was that I was going home.

Mind you, I was not going back without a plan. Conscription was still in force and I really didn't want to join the military. If I could, on medical grounds, get a permanent discharge, I thought, I could both skip the army and get on with being the 'jungle doctor'.

But I had a dilemma, one over which I spent many hours agonising. There were no two ways about it: my discharge plan was based on a lie. But, I asked myself, could ethics be situational? Could a lie be justified if you felt that the system you were facing was evil? I came to the decision that it was. This, and the potential to be part of South Africa's future, justified the lie.

This was the substance underpinning the lie: for a number of years, I had had pain from my back going down into my legs. Such pain, I knew, was probably a spinal tumour or even muscular dystrophy. They say a little knowledge is a dangerous thing but, in reality, a lot of knowledge is far more dangerous. Knowing that I had at least one such debilitating disease, I went in search of confirmation. I underwent scans, bloods, prodding, poking, lumbar punctures and examination of every function and cavity. These produced – nothing ... except that, miraculously, my pain was gone.

The multiple tests had not been in vain, however, for buried in the pile of results was the basis for my plan for medical discharge – a scan that showed I had borderline spinal stenosis, a narrowing of the channel in the spine that carries the spinal cord. A narrowing that can cause pain. Thus armed, I returned to South Africa in January 1990.

In some trepidation, it needs to be said, I marched into the army base with 'spinal stenosis', 'tremendous pain' and 'needing an operation' as my medical excuses for not being fit for purpose. This was my master plan. I thought it was foolproof – only it wasn't. In fact, the South African Defence Force (SADF) was having none of it. Instead of being discharged, I was declared fit for service, but not that fit. I might have succeeded in securing a G3K3 label but it came with a target on my back.

As I think back on the events that have got me here, I realise that I would probably have done the same again, so desperate was I to get home.

WITH AN EXAGGERATED limp, just in case the moon-face corporal is looking, I leave the parade ground and make my way slowly back to the tent that has been my home – mine and 23 other medical graduates – for the last two weeks.

I lift up the tent flap and my eyes adjust to the gloom. The air is stale, musty with the smell of male bodies. It felt hot outside but it's a furnace in here. Two rows of neatly made beds line the canvas walls. In the corner, a tall, bearded, bespectacled figure is reading on his bed. Saul Habiner and I were in med school together. As an Orthodox Jew, his faith means that he is exempt from some training. Since the start of our basic training, Saul has fascinated me. Each morning, while we are all getting dressed, he stands, swaying and praying, a little black box strapped to his head, black tapes around his arms and a prayer shawl around his shoulders. I feel both envious and curious. He seems to have such certainty about his faith and identity. I wonder whether what has forged the identity of this extraordinary people is their belief in their story, authored by God? Has it been the belief, the study and retelling of this story that has helped them keep this identity despite thousands of years of persecution and displacement? I make a mental note to discuss this with Saul. He looks up as I come inside and stand there, immobile. 'You okay?' he asks.

'No.'

'So what's up?' he says. Saul always speaks in a measured way, as if each word is important.

'I've stuffed up,' I say. He puts his book down, waiting for me to go on.

Without really meaning to, I unload the sorry saga of my plan gone awry and my present fears of persecution.

'Ja, that's bad,' he says when my words finally dry up. 'I've seen you taking the gap and I wondered.'

'Wondered what?' I ask. This is not what I want to hear.

'Well, things like you've been in the Jewish line for meals and you're not Jewish,' he says with some concern.

I feel like a naughty schoolboy caught in the act, so I quickly say in my defence, 'Look, I know it's a bit of a stretch but I thought that being half Jewish and with a surname like Japhet, it would be … and the Jewish line is short … about 40 people. Have you seen the other lines? Hundreds!'

'Ja …' Saul is clearly unconvinced, but his tone is kind. 'But it's things like that that will get you into trouble. You need to keep your head down in a place like this.'

'Too late,' I say with a sigh.

But maybe it's not. I have one final examination with a neurosurgeon at 1 Military Hospital this afternoon.

Saul wants to get back to his book, that's obvious, so I leave him and walk slowly to my bed. I can't help marvelling at what is a masterpiece of geometry – the perfect angles of grey blanket meeting white sheets. Who would have believed I could make a bed like that? I flop down onto the masterpiece, hoping vainly for some respite from the heat. The brown tent walls have trapped the morning's warmth, making both thought and movement a chore. Even the omnipresent flies seem to have been grounded. I dip a facecloth in a mug of water and wipe my face before wrapping the cloth around my neck and lying back to gaze at the canvas above me.

I take a few deep breaths, trying to get my emotions under control. The parade ground dust-up has shaken me, but I am also angry. How dare the corporal accuse me of not serving my country? His version of patriotism is not mine. His dream that white people are God-ordained to rule this land is in tatters and I don't think he even knows it. How come guys like him seem so brainwashed, I wonder. Probably because the apartheid government understands what I don't yet – the power of a captivating story. The Afrikaner exodus story, how God led them from religious persecution in Europe to the promised land. Repeat it often enough – the Great Trek, Blood River, 'swart gevaar' and such – and people are willing to live for it. Even die for it. You've got to hand it to them.

Saul's people were victims of a similar narrative propagated by the Nazis. Germans, you are the chosen, the Aryan race. All that is holding you back are the filthy Jews.

But what happens when a dream like that dies? Does life without a purpose, without a big dream, a story to live by, a story to live for, become meaningless? I think it would for me. Perhaps it's in our DNA to believe in a story bigger than ourselves. And if that is so, then we, as a new nation, while remembering our past, will have to craft a story that we all can believe in and work towards. The question is, will I as a white South African be allowed to be part of it? I pray so.

The still air stirs as another varsity friend, 'Ox-eye' Guy, opens the tent flap and shouts, 'Japh! Haven't you left yet? You're going to miss your transport.' Guy is in on my plan. I glance down at my watch. Damn. Missing this appointment would be a stuff-up. I grab my folder of medical notes and scans, thank Saul for the chat as I pass his bed, and hot-foot it towards the parking area. I nimbly dodge some guy ropes and am just rounding the corner of the mess hall when a voice screams 'Japhet!'.

I skid to a halt. I can't believe it. It's the same corporal, his red face a mirror of this morning.

'You can't do press-ups and yet you can run like the devil's behind you – jou bliksem.'

I stutter an excuse. I am in pain … late for an appointment … so sorry.

'Jy krap met 'n kort stokkie aan 'n groot leeu se bal!' he roars. I'm momentarily flummoxed. Something about a lion having me by the balls, I think. 'You're taking chances,' he translates. I am and he knows it. I feel like a rabbit caught in headlights – is my game up? The corporal gazes heavenwards before looking at me. His neck veins deflate and he says quietly, 'Just f… off, Japhet, I don't want to see your face again.'

Gratitude washes over me and this time I am more than happy to comply. I make the bus with seconds to spare.

Still shaken, heart pounding, palms sweaty, I arrive for my appointment with the military neurosurgeon, a big, neat, intense man in his mid-30s. His captain's uniform is freshly pressed; like his office, which is ordered and uncluttered, it seems to be a reflection of his persona.

I feel paralysed by the thought that what happens in the next few minutes could go either way. It's my last chance to get out of here and it feels awful knowing that what I say, like the last witness for the defence, could change everything. The surgeon rises from his desk to greet me. 'Please sit down, Dr Japhet. I've been asked to review your case, so please – tell me your story.'

With all the pathos and medical knowledge I can muster, I proceed to relate the saga of my chronic pain. Most of the time I am speaking the surgeon reads my case notes, occasionally glancing up at me. I sense a growing scepticism and I become more desperate in my narration, the spectre of four more weeks in camp foremost on my mind.

'Okay, let me examine you,' the man says, resignation in his voice.

While I undress, I think to myself that I need to concentrate during the examination, so that I express pain at the appropriate moments. As the surgeon goes about his work, I keep looking at him for clues. Is he buying my story? It's impossible to say. The man is inscrutable. He tells me to get dressed and when I'm back in uniform I go back to his desk where, head bowed, he is writing furiously. After what feels like an age, he leans back in his chair, hands steepled, and gazes at me.

'Dr Japhet,' he begins slowly.

'Yes?' I say, unable to bear the tension.

'After a thorough review of your notes and scans, and after examining you, I can't find any neurological fall-out.' A tingling coldness rushes through my body. 'Apart from a very questionable CT scan, there is no evidence that you have spinal stenosis,' he says with finality.

'But the pain!' I interrupt in desperation with the fearful knowledge that my case is lost.

'Yes, I know,' he continues patiently, 'so this is my recommendation', and he passes me the note.

Resigned, I begin to read. It cites my history and then it gets to the conclusion: 'Diagnosis: long-term pain, symptomatic of spinal stenosis. This will require costly decompression surgery in the near future. Thus, my recommendation is that Private Japhet be classified as G5K5 and released from military service, immediately.'

I do a double-take. '... G5K5 ... released from military service, immediately.' I look up at him. I'm in shock. A flicker of a smile lights up his otherwise impassive face.

4.

BETH SHALOM

The paediatric clinic has been particularly busy this week. We've been swamped by a deluge of newborns with snotty noses and wheezy chests, and worried mothers. It's possibly due to the change of season, but as Sister Theresa points out with a knowing smile, more likely due to the fact that we are nine months post-Christmas.

It's Friday afternoon and you can almost feel the clinic's bustling corridors and crowded rooms let out a collective sigh. Other than the constant traffic in casualty, it will be quiet here until Monday.

Sister Theresa scurries around the clinic, sorting stray files and tidying the familiar flotsam and jetsam of abandoned dummies, spilt milk and safety-pins. 'I hope you have a good weekend, Garth.' She chuckles. 'Maybe next week will be easier.'

'I hope so for your sake, Sister,' I respond. 'Remember I'm away next week … on a retreat …?'

'Of course – I remember now,' she says. Then, putting her hand on mine, she says sincerely, 'I will pray for you.'

As I say the word 'retreat' I'm suddenly jolted by how properly weird this is. Maybe the industrial dosages I'm taking of my head medicine are messing with my brain, but somehow I have committed to this 'time out'. I am going for a full week to meet people and a God I don't really know, and I'm going to ask them to help me make some sense of my life.

It was my pastor, Andrew Luke, who suggested the retreat centre in Hilton. To say that I wasn't particularly enamoured with the idea would be an understatement. My imagination had immediately conjured up visions of austere monks, their long periods of silent prayer made possible by great bladder control. I hope I'm wrong. But my internal battle with questions of meaning, purpose and direction never seems to let up, so I have decided to give the retreat a try. What have I got to lose?

Later that afternoon, I descend into the KwaZulu-Natal Midlands. Despite the trauma that I've experienced here, it's still my happy place, my soul place, so, despite my apprehension, I have a lightness of spirit that lifts even more as I enter the comforting blanket of mist, synonymous with the Hilton area.

It's dark by the time I reach Beth Shalom, the retreat centre run by Jim and Heather Johnson, both of whom are originally from Northern Ireland. This centre is the realisation of their dream to create a beautiful place of rest for people to commune with God, themselves and nature.

On arrival I am welcomed by the 'eep, eep, eep' of fruit bats swooping in the sky – and by Jim himself. On the phone, with his lilting Irish accent, he had sounded sage-like, and so he is in person: a wiry man in late middle age with sparkling blue eyes set in a weather-worn face. Beside him is Heather. She envelops me in a warm hug, takes my hand and welcomes me into their rambling house. 'Ah, famished you must be, Garth? I hope you are, as I've a wee bit of dinner prepared for you,' she says, directing me to a table set for one.

'Aren't you going to join me?' I say, panic in my voice.

'No, no, laddie,' Jim responds. 'You just quieten down, settle in and when you're finished eating, we'll chat.'

And so I eat a solitary dinner. No book, TV, music or conversation. It is an uncomfortable experience. Afterwards I join Jim in his book-lined study. I sit expectantly. I wonder how this is going to pan out.

'Have you ever spent time meditating on God's word?' Jim asks.

'Uh, not really,' I admit.

'It's like studying poetry. You take a piece and wrestle with it. You look for patterns and for meaning, which are often not obvious at first reading.'

He pauses. 'You with me?' he asks. I think I am, so he continues. 'This week I want you to spend time with Psalm 139. I think it's one of the most beautiful.'

The psalm may be beautiful, but I also know it's short. 'Just Psalm 139?' I ask.

'Yes.' Jim smiles.

A whole week of silent meal-times and only a page to read. What is this? I am going to be driven further up the wall.

'I also want you to write down your story,' Jim continues after a long pause.

'My story?' I ask sceptically.

'Yes. If we don't spend time reflecting on where we have come from, it's difficult to see where we are going.' Finally Jim is sounding more sage-like. He looks at me enquiringly and I give him a humourless smile.

'Well, that will be fun,' I say. 'If the next 27 years are like the last 27, I think I may want out.'

'Believe me, Garth, understanding your own story is one of the greatest gifts you can give yourself and, in time, others too. It is, I believe, the foundation for healing.' He can probably see I'm not convinced, so he says. 'Trust me with this, Garth. And trust God.'

I'm not sure I trust either of them.

'Start as far back as your memory goes,' Jim continues. 'Try to capture the events of your life and the feelings that accompanied them. Don't worry about your language or structure. Just write.'

I shift uncomfortably in my chair. 'And that's it?'

'Aye, that's all. We'll spend about half an hour together each day to see how you're going, but otherwise it's between you and God. Heather and I will be praying for you.'

I am horrified and Jim can tell.

'I can see you are anxious, my lad,' he says kindly. 'This can be scary. To stop all our doing and just be for a change. But don't you worry, you'll soon settle in. Sit in the garden, go for walks, eat slowly, sleep. Try to use all your senses. I think you're going to be surprised.'

I walk to my bedroom with a leaden heart. What a let-down. I had expected to come here and have some wise guru unravel the tangled threads of my life, not this. How on earth am I going to fill this week? If I had a case of Stuffed Head Syndrome (SHS) before I arrived, I will be certifiable by the time I leave.

I HAVE ALWAYS loved arriving at places in the dark. When I was child, at Christmas time I used to sneak into the lounge when everyone else was asleep and try to guess what was hidden under the wrapping paper of all the presents beneath the tree. This feels the same, the anticipation of what the light of morning will bring.

I wake early and with the dawn I feel my spirits lift. I walk out into the garden. It's fresh outside and last night's mist has left a sheen that will burn off during the day. A tennis court-sized kikuyu lawn is protected from the road by a line of tall pine trees, edged by flower-beds. This is not an ordered garden, however, but one where a profusion of shrubs, plants and trees are engaged in a never-ending friendly wrestle with the gardener. A huge avo tree stands squarely in the middle of the grass, lord of all it surveys. Scents and cabbage butterflies waft over the garden. And then there is colour, lots of it, greens, blues, pinks, whites and reds that seem to change hue with the shifting clouds.

Do I take this in all at once? No, I do not.

As a doctor, my life is subject to the tyranny of time: the shrill of the alarm that starts the day, then shift on, meal break, shift off, punctuated by the constant refrain of 'We need you immediately, doctor.' There is a comfort in this. I don't usually have time to think, let alone observe.

But here I have been given a gift. Not that I appreciate it initially. I'm driven up the wall – or, to be more precise, the avo tree, the road, the pool, as I climb, walk, run, swim. Anything to kill time between meals. But then, like the Duracell Bunny's companion, the one with the no-name batteries, I start to slow down.

I find myself doing weird things like sitting watching a collection of flowering bushes for what might be hours. For the first time in my life, I actually look at a flower. Not like the quick glance I've given to flowers bought for an evening's date, but really looking. A cluster of delicate red stamens peer out from a ruff of purple and red leaves. Bees and glossy green malachite sunbirds compete for the flowers' nectar. Jim tells me they're fuchsias. I begin to appreciate the perfection of the shape, colour, scent and the rhythm of nature. I begin to appreciate the artist behind it.

This is all good – slowing down, sleeping, seeing more, eating slowly – but I'm struggling on two fronts. I read and re-read Psalm 139 and it's nice, but so is ice-cream. There are no Aha! moments. I'm also struggling to write. Each time I sit down, it feels like there is another flower to watch or tree to climb. Or maybe I just don't want to go there.

'HOW ARE YOU doing, laddie?' Jim says as we sit down for our daily half-hour. 'Still finding it hard?'

On previous days I've told Jim where I'm at, hoping he will give me a new reading and release me from this writing thing, but to no avail. This guru is not for moving. I give him a despairing look.

'Stick with the psalm, Garth, and don't you be agonising over it,' Jim soothes. 'I didn't just randomly select it, laddie. I believe that there is meaning in there for you.'

I sigh. I tell Jim I'll keep going with the psalm, but what about my story? I'm finding writing my story almost impossible.

'Ah yes, your story,' Jim says. 'Many of us struggle to write our stories, but it's one of the most valuable things a person can ever do.' He slips into sage mode. 'We can't change the past but we can change how it affects us and who it makes us. It may not seem that how you tell your story is important, even if it's just to yourself, but how you interpret your life and tell its story can have profound effects on your future and the person you become. And I want to urge you to look for the positives in the hard times you may have been through. I think that you'll find looking at your life like that uplifting.'

As before, I remain sceptical but I promise to try. Jim rises and puts his hand on my shoulder. 'You'll be all right, you will. Just make a start – and don't shy away from the difficult bits.'

I compromise. I climb the avo tree but take an exercise book and pen with me. I manage to procrastinate further by searching for the ideal spot, but eventually I begin. Taking Jim's advice, I don't try too hard. I just recall images and scenes from my past and I patch them together. The more I write, the more I remember and the more uncomfortable I feel. There are happy times but it's the tough times that are the most vivid. My gut lurches and my heart responds.

I recall the sheer panic I experienced whenever my mother left me. The irrational fears of the dark, of abandonment, of illness, of everything. The shame I felt as I dropped out of one school after another, and the feelings of hopelessness and despair that overwhelmed me as my 'Jungle Doctor' dreams shattered.

I had thought, before climbing the tree, that I was making good progress towards a Zen-like state. Now I just feel raw. But it's a different sort of raw. As a doctor I know that when a wound refuses to heal, the best approach is often to open it up, strip out all the gunk and expose fresh tissue. Maybe that's what this is.

The rumble of afternoon thunder followed by a loud crack grounds me quickly into the present. Being ignited by a bolt of lightning will not be pretty so I clamber hastily down the tree. As I make a bee-line for the house, the storm breaks. The garden, which moments before had been a vision of tranquillity, is transformed by the downpour. Large drops of rain bounce off leaves and wind screams through branches. I love storms. There is something wild and cleansing about them. They've always given me the urge to take off my clothes and dance. And so I do.

The rain sets in, greying out the garden and for the next day consigning me to a different space – my room. I sit in a chair, the soft thrumming on the roof and the drip-drip of the leaves providing a backdrop for my thoughts. With less panic and more understanding I return to my own story, to read and re-read it.

It feels in a way like turning a tapestry over. Where before I was just seeing the nonsensical tangled threads of my life, I begin to see patterns emerge.

Then, with the force of an unexpected wave, an insight crashes into me. Sure I was a nursery, primary and high school dropout, but that was more due to my mother's unspoken signals of 'I need you' than my own weakness.

Suddenly I am angry. I stand up and pace. I'm angry at my mother. She had fed my insecurity and reinforced my anxiety. Why? Why had she done this to me?

'Garth, darling, please be careful when you play soccer today.'

'Are you coming to watch, Mum?'

'No, darling, I couldn't bear to see you get hurt.'

Cot-sides at five.

Every precious hair on my head needed to be protected. I mean this literally. While all the other children went under the vicious blades of the school barber, Garth had a letter from his mother insisting that his hair be cut by her hairdresser.

I am *so* pissed off. Not only am I angry at my mother, but also at my dad. Why did he not step in and stand up for me, give me the confidence to get hurt and bounce back? Where was he when Mum was protecting my hair like it was some exotic bush?

But for the first time I begin to feel another emotion too. Pride. Not in a boastful way, but pride in, despite setbacks, having achieved much. Anxiety, fear of blood, not great at maths and science, a seriously hard time at medical school and yet here I am: Dr Japhet. I had set my heart on a course and stayed with it, even if it was the wrong course for me.

Then I have a reality check. Part of my reason for doing medicine was because I thought that Dr Japhet would be more attractive than Mr Japhet and yet, apart from a psycho nurse who used to stalk me and do things like leave a light bulb outside my door with a note saying 'You are the light of my life', my dreams on that front are definitely just that, dreams!

But still, a sense is building within me that my course was no accident.

For the first time I'm eager to chat to Jim.

'So, laddie, I sense a change in you. Did you make a start on your story then?'

I smile and describe my time to him. I leave out the bit about dancing in the rain, though, for fear he might call for immediate psychiatric back-up.

'I'm so grateful, lad. I've been praying for this breakthrough. I'm constantly amazed at how powerful reviewing our own stories can be. It's an opportunity to understand, affirm and, if necessary, forgive our younger selves and others. And, often, to see God's hand in our lives. I believe you will be leaving this place changed.'

Jim tells me to stick with writing my story, but reminds me to set aside some time for the psalm. 'There is richness there, there is,' he says.

I step into the garden with a sense of anticipation. How I've changed in these few days. Instead of dashing to a destination, this time I amble. Sunlight transforms a wet spider's web into a prism, radiating colour. A hadeda bashes its nose into the damp earth; a few futile stabs and then a brown thread wiggles from its beak and disappears. Flowers glisten, the moisture covering their petals making their colours seem hyper-real.

All very beautiful but also very wet. Where am I going to sit?

At the top of the garden is a large yesterday, today and tomorrow bush in full bloom. I remember Dad teaching me that on the first day (yesterday) the flowers are purple, the second day (today) they change to a pastel lavender and on the third day (tomorrow) they change to an almost white colour. And then they die. Strangely, there is a dry patch under the bush just big enough for me to sit in. Definitely a God-incidence, I think. This is where I am meant to sit. The bush is a symbol, a sign! Then I catch myself. Maybe it's no such thing; maybe it's just a patch that happens to be dry because of the slant at which the rain was falling. Either way, I sit down. The scent from the bush is overwhelming.

I open my Bible to Psalm 139. I read it for the umpteenth time. Perhaps the time I have spent with my own story changes my perception because verses that had previously just been poetic text now jump out at me.

> [8] If I go up to the heavens, you are there;
> if I make my bed in the depths, you are there.
> [9] If I rise on the wings of the dawn,
> if I settle on the far side of the sea,
> [10] even there your hand will guide me,
> your right hand will hold me fast.

My life has been largely underpinned by fear. Fear of abandonment. These verses shout out, 'You will never be abandoned. No matter where you go and what you do, I will not only care for you, I will guide you.' It may sound a bit dramatic, but I suddenly know that this is true.

My reverie is momentarily distracted by the rattle of a lawnmower starting up. The sun is out and I see Jim, stripped to the waist, in the distance. Clearly monk-like living is good for the body as well as the soul. The scent of freshly cut kikuyu wafts over me and my mind wanders.

My thoughts are interrupted by the incessant call of a Piet-my-vrou, the red-chested cuckoo, and I squint up into the tree where the sound is coming from. They're very shy birds and seldom seen, but I see him – his little russet chest, flitting from branch to branch. This is definitely another sign … and maybe it is, because I'm suddenly struck by the thought: If I were to ask this bird, 'Who is responsible for this garden?' he might chirp, 'The gardener, of course. He is the only one who understands this garden. We Piet-my-vrous, we just do what Piet-my-vrous were created to do, no more no less.' Then he'd hit me with this parting shot: 'And perhaps you should too.'

This revelation feels like a big deal. Stop trying to change the whole world. Be what He created you for. Then my inner voice mumbles, 'Good insight, Garth. And what might that be?' What indeed?

The mower grumbles to a halt. A sweaty Jim calls over to me, disturbing my thoughts. 'Time for our session it is, laddie. The last one, if my memory serves me correctly.'

I can't believe I've been here a whole week. I could easily stay for another.

A FRESHLY SHOWERED Jim sits opposite me in his study. I am in my usual leather-backed chair. We look at each other and then Jim says, 'Questions, laddie?'

'Yes – quite a few,' I say.

Jim waits for me to go on.

'This has been nothing like I thought it would be. I expected to leave here with my questions answered and with a direct line to God.'

Jim chuckles as if I have said something really amusing. 'Not this side of heaven, lad.'

'Yes, I know that now, and I think I feel more at peace with the understanding that life is a mystery to be lived, not understood.'

'Very poetic, Garth.'

'Not original, but true,' I smile. 'I came here being really at sea about my life. But I feel that, through this time, God has affirmed me, that nothing is lost. I am more certain that He has created me for a purpose and will use both the good and bad times.' I pause. 'Except I'm not yet sure what that purpose is?'

Jim leans forward and takes both my hands in his. 'You've driven on the roads around here when the mist has been so thick you can't see more than a car's length ahead of you?'

'Often,' I say.

'And the only way you can steer is by following the cats' eyes in the road?' I nod. 'Well, so it is with life, laddie. All you need to do is look for the next cat's eye in the road. God has already written your story. He knows your purpose. Even though it may be all misty to you, just trust Him and take the next step.'

I sit for a moment in contemplation.

'So I don't need to have the full picture to know my purpose?'

'Not at all, my lad. Just be open to the next step, to the next step is all.'

'But if the mist is so thick that I can't see a thing, no cats' eyes, nothing? What then? A step into the void?'

'No, laddie. Then we wait, knowing in His good time that the mist will lift enough for your next step.'

'Okay,' I say slowly, 'so best I be getting back to the clinic then?'

'Indeed you must,' Jim says. His gaze moves from me to the window and I follow it. 'Can't see much,' he says, his eyes crinkling in amusement.

'Thick mist,' I say.

'And that's okay?' he asks.

'Yes.'

And it is.

IN OTHERS' WORDS ...

Many of those I interviewed in researching the material for this book brought up the importance of knowing and appreciating their family's stories, particularly as it allowed them insight and ownership of their own.

As a journalist and writer, Ufrieda Ho believed she was 'born to tell other people's stories'. It was only when she put pen to paper to write her memoir, *Paper Sons and Daughters: Growing up Chinese in South Africa*, that she began to unpack her own story. She already knew the power of story, coming from a tradition of oral storytelling down generations, and she was an avid reader as a child. But in exploring themes of identity and belonging as she traced the path her immigrant family took to South Africa and examined the community in which she was raised, she mined deeper levels of understanding. She has a strong interest in anthropology and generational connectivity – 'We are threaded together with stories of those who came before us,' was the way she described these connections to me. 'Sharing your story gives shape to our evolving identity.'

Researching the informal illegal gambling activity known as *fahfee* in the Chinese community in which she grew up, and in which her father was involved but which was never talked about, unlocked some deep and painful but ultimately empowering emotions for Ufrieda. Others with similar backdrops to their family stories felt that she had given voice to their stories and many reached out to her to say this after her book was published. 'Being able to identify with a story,' Ufrieda said, 'and I don't mean just mine, validates your feelings.'

Debbie Kirsten came to owning her own story after a somewhat circuitous route. First as the daughter of a well-known political activist and

Christian leader Michael Cassidy, and then marrying into a famous cricketing family, there was a time when she didn't believe that anyone really wanted to get to know her for her own sake. 'I thought my story was insignificant,' she said. From being a freelance travel writer as she toured the world with her husband Gary, and then as a columnist for a Christian magazine, she gradually realised that that was not true. People related to her. Her 'ordinary' stories of life, motherhood, travelling, and the importance of her Christian faith resonated with many. Still, when she was approached by a publisher to write a book, she struggled to find the way in. Something inside her told her it was her own story she needed to write – 'Yes, it might sit in this massive story of cricket' – and finally, through prayer, reflection and reading others' stories, the breakthrough came: 'Use your own voice and tell your own story.' The book that resulted, *Chai Tea and Ginger Beer*, touched many people's lives. It also drew Debbie further into the power of owning and telling your own story. It led her to research and devise a course for other 'ordinary people' to do the same, based on 'owning the shape of your story'. This begins with a practical exercise: mapping a graph with the high and low points in your life, the mountains and the valleys, and then flipping the graph, so that the valleys become mountains and vice versa. 'It's about perspective,' Debbie explained in our interview. 'If we change our perspective, we can see triumph in having lived through a hard time rather than failure.'

Wits academic Laura Dison, who co-ordinates the post-graduate diploma in Higher Education, understands the value of being better able to know who you are when you know the stories of those who came before you. Like Ufrieda, she came from a migrant family – in her case they were refugees from Lithuania – and her parents were of a generation who did not easily talk about personal things. 'There was always that strong need to know where they came from,' she acknowledged. As someone whose students are being trained to be educators, she was pleased to discover 'a thread of education in my family, my grandmother, aunts and cousins'. It was affirming. 'It's nice to feel like part of a tradition,' she said. Much of

Laura's focus in the academic sphere is on teaching, mentoring and helping students and colleagues developmentally through writing. Although she hasn't written extensively about her own personal story, she did spend time writing about her sister, who died young, an activity she experienced as cathartic – 'interviewing people and finding out that she was a remarkable person. She was a lawyer and although she died at a young age, she had already accomplished a lot. I looked at some of the work she did on human rights. Fascinating things emerged around her. She was also disabled and had polio when she was three years old, so it was a lot of stuff around that as well. Some of those stories made me closer to her but also helped me have a better understanding of myself and how I fitted in.'

One of South Africa's most acclaimed advertising, marketing and strategy gurus is Ivan Moroke. Currently the CEO of Kantar SA, the global consulting and research firm, he enjoyed a successful career leading advertising agencies and marketing strategy firms and industry bodies. He was the first person to recognise the value of what would become the Heartlines' 'What's Your Story?' campaign. (He is also the chair of the Heartlines board.) In our interview he acknowledged that his backstory is not an unusual one for a black child in South Africa: brought up by a single mother in a township, in his case Atteridgeville, Pretoria, during apartheid. But it was his mother's fierce love, her resilience and the value she attached to education and knowledge that did much to shape his future. I asked him how looking to his past and sharing his personal story had helped him looking forward.

'It is like writing a book,' he said. 'If you are still alive after writing a book, you have got a perspective about your life now based on where you have been and that then influences how you view going forward. There might be some things that were blind spots before you shared your story, or wrote the book, but they are not blind spots anymore. So in your future, you are going to deal with those things differently because you are aware of them.'

Professor Jimmy Volmink might be the Dean of the Faculty of Medicine and Health Sciences at Stellenbosch University today, but he, like Ivan, came from humble beginnings. Understanding, owning and sharing his story, he believes, have shaped his life. During apartheid South Africa and growing up in the 70s in Athlone in the Cape, it was his hardworking parents – his father a labourer who went to work on his bicycle; his mother the 'tea girl' for an oil company – who instilled in him and his siblings the values they carried with them and lived by. 'My mother told me: "Be proud of what you do, whether it is sweeping the street or something else. Always do your best."'

When Jimmy was a medical student in his final years of study, apartheid South Africa forbade doctors who were not white examining patients in the white wards in teaching hospitals. This harsh reality was brought starkly home to him when a patient he'd been asked to take blood from refused to be touched by him and called for a white doctor. 'Do you know who I am?' the man said to the young med student. 'I was an interpreter in the Steve Biko case. And I am so glad he got what he deserved. I am so glad his life ended that way.' Prof Volmink held this story in his head for many years, including the fact that his superior just laughed the incident off and did not challenge the patient's attitude. 'We often do not take time to really process what is happening at the time,' Prof Volmink said. 'It can be many years later, when you reflect back, that you start getting angry about it. You realise what happened to your parents, what happened to you, your family and so on. I think the processing sometimes comes much later.'

Another South African who grew up in challenging circumstances is Quinton Pretorius. His formative years were spent in a volatile family, where alcohol and tempestuous emotions could cause violent havoc and fear. Book learning did not come easily to him but he discovered that he had a natural talent when it came to the spoken word. Today he is in high demand as a speaker on multiple platforms across many disciplines. One thing he is sure of: he knows the personal power of owning his story and also the power of sharing it. 'Once we start understanding our story and understand the impact of those events in our lives, we can then proactively begin to re-engage it,' he told me. It took him a long time to inhabit his story, which includes sexual abuse at the hands of a friend's father in primary school, the violent death of his dad during an altercation in a shop, mental and verbal abuse from a jealous stepfather, and the bewildering withdrawal of affection on the part of his mother.

Like Quinton, it wasn't easy for pastor Steven Mzee to acknowledge and come to terms with his childhood in Nairobi, which was one of poverty and struggle. His single mother entrusted his care to his grandmother, a cleaner at a hospital, and they lived in Kibera, one of the largest and most densely populated and under-serviced slums on the continent. His grandmother's strictness and not always physically demonstrated love kept him only narrowly on the straight and narrow and there were many times when he found himself veering towards a life of crime, and the bitter seductions of alcohol and drugs. Denying the reality of his childhood circumstances was something Steven carried with him into his adult life. 'I had always blocked my past ... I did not want to hear about or be reminded of it.' It was only years later that he found the courage to absorb his past and to share his personal story in his preaching. He told me it was one of the most powerful things he had ever done; it transformed the relationship with his congregation from him being a respected but distant figure to a fellow journeyer who, like them, had lived.

Jonathan Robinson is the CEO and founder of award-winning Bean There fair trade coffee. He understood the effectiveness of learning and understanding through story from his pastor father, Leigh, who used story in his preaching. It was also through hearing his parents talk openly and honestly about their lives before they met and also about their at times rocky marriage – they married when Jonathan was two years old, shortly after his birth mother had died tragically in a car accident – that he realised the importance of owning his own story. 'My parents demonstrated to me how important it is to be vulnerable,' he told me. 'Not hold it all in and pretend that everything is perfect. When you mess up, own up to it. Being vulnerable, apologising, owning and being able to share how you messed up is powerful. The moment someone looks like they are too good to be true, they usually are. It is only once they say, "These are my struggles. These are my challenges. This is where I have fallen down. I wanted to end my life …" When you hear that from your father, suddenly he becomes human.'

Zolani Mahola, former lead singer of Freshlyground, is a storyteller who can command an audience with her voice and music, but not many know her full story. It wasn't until relatively recently, she said, that she was able to talk to her father about the death of her mother. She was only six years old when her mother died – in childbirth – and the family moved away immediately after the funeral. No one talked about her mother; no one ever explained to the little girl what had happened. Even now her father finds it difficult to talk about the woman who was the love of his life. It was having her own children that made Zolani want to know more about herself, to know her own story. Her song 'Nomvula' is written for her parents. It is in Xhosa and begins with the words: 'Come closer, my friend, here is a long tale …' 'People may not understand the words,' Zolani said, 'but something is transferred in the mood. It's the song that always resonates the most.' When it comes to owning your story and the things that have shaped it, Zolani is candid: 'You are unique. You are the only person who can tell your particular story. So you do have a story to tell, just by virtue that you are.'

Olefile Masangane, one of my Heartlines colleagues and a friend, was raised by a single mother. For a while as a child he was given to believe that his father was dead, until people in the community kept saying how much he looked like his father, even walked like him, and he confronted his mother, who told him the truth. It made him an angry teenager. Although he did manage to forge some sort of relationship with his father, it was his older brother who was a strong and positive role model for him. In researching his family as an adult, Olefile began to understand better the powerful influence of antecedents on subsequent generations – not only where you come from but who you come from.

Gcina Mhlophe, probably South Africa's most famous storyteller, began to explore and try to understand her dual identities – Zulu on her paternal side; Xhosa on her mother's – after her mother's death when she wrote her award-winning play *Have You Seen Zandile?* Through the process of writing it and then performing it, which she has done many times all over the world, she was able to finally own her personal story. It is important at a significant stage in one's life, she told me, to 'create a space and look back'.

Someone who understands the challenges of identity and belonging is Irene Robinson. Of Danish heritage, her parents emigrated to Canada when she was a child. 'My dad was a bit of a maverick,' Irene told me, 'taking his wife and two small children, and sailing to Canada, not knowing any English at all. My mom, being an introvert and also not knowing the language, and with no support in this new country, seemed to live a rather isolated life.' Irene remembers those years as being tough, with her parents trying to get work wherever they could, and very little money coming in. 'If I think of my childhood,' she reflected, 'what comes most to mind is that we had to figure out how to survive.' Because of this, the family moved around a lot, with Irene going to a number of different schools, and with it a sense of displacement, of often starting over. Questions from other children like 'Why do you look so different?', 'Why do you talk so funny?' were constantly thrown at her. 'And then, when I finished high school, my mother said, "Okay, I've done my part, now it's your time to go." I packed my suitcase, got on a Greyhound bus, and left our little town and went into the city of Calgary and looked for a job and a place to live.'

Not all of us have the perceived luxury of taking time to reflect, to go within, to first tell their story to themselves before fully owning it and being able to share it. It is not an easy process. It can be uncomfortable, painful even, as I discovered at Beth Shalom, but out of it will come understanding and compassion, for the child you once were and, hopefully, for those who came before you.

PART 2

FRAMING – THE RICHES OF IMAGINATION, THE POVERTY OF ASSUMPTION

For years I have been aware of just what a powerful influence story has had on me. My childhood was awash with story. My mother read to me constantly, picture books, fables, myth and adventure stories. When I could read myself, I immersed myself in books, which could transport and transform me and allowed my imagination to spark and sizzle and a young boy's mind to dream and aspire to performing seemingly impossible feats.

As a child who was often alone, the companionship of the radio and its dramatised stories, plays and series kept me riveted for hours. Oral storytelling, with all of the embellishment of voice, tone, gesture and moments of suspense, can hold an audience captive like nothing else. Later on, films and television held my attention and it wasn't long before I developed a love for theatre and plays performed on stage before a live audience. Stories are framed in so many ways. The well-chosen words of an exquisitely crafted haiku verse or a few short lines of homespun wisdom penned by someone newly literate can have as powerful an effect as a novel the length and depth of *War and Peace*. Song lyrics are often powerful stories set to music getting us to potentially think and feel differently.

Although I was keenly aware that stories shaped my thinking and my life, what I was unaware of was that I was living my own story and that how I chose to tell it to myself and others could profoundly affect my mental well-being and indeed my future.

Well told, fact or fiction, stories have more power to shape humanity than any weapon or virus known to man. It is through telling stories that we pass on wisdom from one generation to the next. It is the stories that we have embraced about our families, our ethnicities and countries that shape the way we see ourselves and the world, and how we think and act. They teach us what our society considers acceptable behaviour and what will not be forgiven. Stories connect us to one another and enable us to empathise, allowing us to feel what it's like to walk in someone else's shoes.

As I recount in Part 2, it was a story I read as a child that captured my imagination and made me believe that an unlikely future was possible.

For story to work its magic, however, it first has to be told, listened to and heard.

Like most people, I have made snap assumptions about others before they've had a chance to tell their stories. I have been guilty of making assumptions based on my unconscious or learned bias – basing my assumptions on, among other things, a person's race, gender, age, ethnicity. When we stereotype each other we are the poorer for the casual laziness of accepted, unchallenged views, the received 'truisms' untested or tried. Some of these assumptions are harmless but many are deeply wounding and lead to the divisions and mistrust that plague our society.

I have had a number of encounters that have brought home to me the danger of assumption and that have helped me to try to do better and to understand more fully. Some of these encounters I recount here in Part 2 and the learnings I took away from them have, I hope, made me more intentional about getting to know a person's story and not let a false assumption be a stumbling block.

Some of those people I interviewed for this book spoke powerfully to the theme of how stories, differently framed, differently delivered and imaginatively constructed, can make a lasting impact – even change lives. Our brains are wired for story in way that no other creature's is. In the same way that a mood-altering drug affects thought and action so can and does story. While a drug can momentarily alter our perception of reality, stories can inspire us to imagine a new reality for ourselves. They inspire us to dream of what the story of our lives may look like.

5.

EMERALD ISLE

Is there anything worse than feeling seasick? I'm sure there is, but right now nothing comes to mind. What does come to mind, however, is whether I'm going to make it to the bathroom in time before I am violently ill in public. Death feels appealing.

Taking a ferry from France to Ireland seemed like both a fine and a cheap plan – on dry land, that was – and my chance to be on a ship, even if only for a night. It's 1985, I'm 21 years old and backpacking solo through Europe. This trip is all about adventure, right? Right. But a storm snatching up a big ship like this and flinging it around like a cork was not part of my adventure reckoning.

Everything is moving, creaking. Maybe we are sinking, but what of it? Right now I couldn't care less. I feel like I'm in a giant pin-ball machine, being flipped from one side to the other. I crash painfully into the steel walls as I stagger down the passage. My nausea is compounded by the stench of diesel and musty carpets. I'm almost there. I lunge for the door, stagger to the toilet, grab the edges of the welcoming bowl and eject the remains of a ridiculously expensive sandwich. That really hurt. I'm a student on a very tight budget.

I lurch back into the passageway and slowly make my way towards the cabins. I'm making some progress when, on rounding a corner, I walk slap-bang into a stockily built man.

'So sorry,' I stutter.

'No harm done,' the man says, grinning broadly. His sweaty red face is framed by an unruly fuzz of dark hair. He looks at me quizzically. 'You okay, lad?' he asks.

I nod and smile weakly.

'You don't look too good, do ye? Have you got a bad dose of something?' He gives me a knowing wink and a jovial slap on the shoulder, which makes me stagger.

The man's Irish accent is so thick I can hardly work out what he is saying, but I presume he's asking me if I'm infectious or drunk.

'I'm fine, thanks,' I say. 'Just seasick.'

The Irishman is clearly feeling a lot finer than me. 'Ah, we can't have that then, can we?' he says. 'Not with a whole night ahead of us.'

I'm a little bemused, but before I can say anything else he says, 'You come with me now, boyo.' And with that he grasps me firmly by the elbow and steers me back the way I've come. 'I make this trip every week and there is only one cure for what ails you. It's the black stuff, the Guinness.'

To be honest, he could have offered me anything right then – snake oil, cocaine, lizard blood, anything – and I'd have taken it. With the storm raging outside and my guts still churning inside, I become a willing recipient of his Irish medicine.

I am not a drinker – although not for lack of trying. It's just that I am inherently incapable of sustained drinking. After only a few drinks, I am either violently ill or I fall asleep. But tonight is different. I join Dylan, for that is his name, and three of his mates at the ferry bar. They, like Dylan, seem completely unaffected by the ship's motion and they welcome me like a long-lost friend.

'You're from Africa then, are you?' Nolan asks.

'Yes, I am.'

Nolan looks at me through glazed eyes. 'So, then you're one of those albino types?'

'Uh, no ...' I stammer, taken aback.

He squints, moving closer to take a look at me, a confused expression on his face. 'But you're from Africa, you say, and yet you're not black.' His tone is smug; he is sure of his knowledge of the world.

Dylan raises his eyes heavenwards. 'Will you listen to yourself?' he says. 'Don't be a complete eejit, Nolan, don't you read your papers?'

Nolan looks puzzled. 'Course I do,' he says.

'Looking at page three girls in *The Sun* doesn't count as reading, you wally,' Dylan says with a grin. 'If you'd really been reading, you'd know that there are white people in Africa.' Nolan gives an embarrassed shrug and Dylan moves swiftly on. 'Let's start you with a wee whiskey dram,' he says, indicating two fingers to the barman. 'Nothing like it to settle the stomach.'

Encouraged by my new 'friends', I take a gulp of the amber liquid. Fire! I cough and splutter, evoking a tide of laughter, glass-clinking and back-slapping. I'm beginning to think that beyond any altruism in helping me, Dylan and company are looking forward to getting me wasted. Whatever their motivation, the whiskey followed by a few pints of 'the black stuff' works! It feels that instead of fighting the swaying of the ship we are both able to move in unison. I no longer want to die.

The rest of the night passes in a haze.

Morning finally dawns. I'm not feeling seasick now, just sick sick. I've a pounding headache and eyes that feel like I've been through a sand storm. Amazingly, my friends look fine.

'Well, you're looking a bit knackered, lad. You were as full as a bingo bus on a Friday evenin', you were,' Dylan says.

'I was?'

'Yes, drunk, lad. Drunk. Now let's get you something to eat. Line the stomach with something greasy. Then you'll feel as right as rain.'

While Nolan goes off to find 'something greasy', Dylan summons me on deck. 'Fresh air will do you good and it's a beautiful day to be arriving in Rosslare,' he says as he guides me out of the bar.

I stagger out into the sunshine, squinting painfully. The sea is calm, the wind has dropped. Like a baby smiling after a torrid night, you would never had guessed there had been a storm. On the horizon, growing slowly larger, is a ripple of green hills and a smudge of buildings that I guess to be the port. As we approach, the land comes into focus. I see a patchwork of variegated green fields, with patches of scrub, rolling down to a sandy bay. It's beautiful.

I'm feeling much better, thanks to the salt air and the greasy 'banger' sandwich that Nolan thrusts into my hand. 'So, boyo, where are you off to?' Dylan asks.

I tell him I'm planning to take a bus to Waterford, where I'll stay in a youth hostel. Nolan nods sagely. 'Beautiful place, Waterford. Great pubs with some of the best craic in the district.'

Seeing my eyes widen, Dylan chuckles. 'The word's "craic", lad, not "crack"! It's the word we use for music and fun. If a pub's got great craic, then there'll be live music, good food and, if you're lucky, lad, some fine Irish lasses.'

As the ferry eases into port we make our way back inside. I pick up my rucksack and say my goodbyes. I am so grateful to these men who have shepherded me on this crossing and who have, unknowingly, birthed in me a love of the Irish. As I leave the ferry and head towards the bus station, I suddenly realise that I haven't paid for anything. I turn on my heel and rush back to the boat, frantically looking for a familiar face, but my friends are long gone.

It's mid-morning when I arrive in Waterford, feeling mildly shaken. Having just survived wanting to die on the ferry in a vicious storm – and now certain that I *don't* want to die – the bus trip almost took matters out of my hands. We had careered through impossibly narrow lanes, the driver seemingly oblivious to any possibility of oncoming traffic and, when there inevitably was, through some sort of sixth sense, somehow always managing to swerve at just the right time. When I wasn't praying or covering my eyes, what I had seen of the land, through spread fingers, was stunning.

It's the greenness that strikes me most. The Emerald Isle is truly well named. Everything is green – the hedges that line the lanes, the trees, and then the grass! The grass is almost luminous in its brilliance. Perhaps it strikes me so deeply because of the contrast with the greens of home, greens that always seem to have some space for a little brown. Not here. This country is green like I have never seen before.

Waterford is Ireland's oldest city and port, dating back to AD 853. It is an eclectic mixture of Ireland through the ages. It was my mother who had suggested I visit Waterford for the famous crystal. Not the healing sort, but beautiful cut glass. So, with no real plan and seeing that it was close to Rosslare, I have ended up here.

Smart new buildings and run-down shops and homes sit cheek by jowl with remnants of the city's Viking and medieval past. Leaving the bus stop, I wander around the town while I'm waiting for the hostel to open at 3pm. I am properly tired. The blue skies of the early morning have been replaced by scudding walls of grey cloud and intermittent rain. I find a small café to hang out in till opening time. I've perfected the art of nursing a coffee and avoiding waiters' scowls. My best time so far is over two hours.

Eventually, just before 3pm I make my way to The Portree youth hostel. It's an unimposing three-storeyed building looking onto a busy street in the centre of the town. I walk up the steps and am greeted by the kind of reception common to most hostels: a desk staffed by students much the same age as me and on the walls notice-boards with hostel rules, tour offers, entertainment options and, importantly, where to find cheap food and drink.

'Single or sharing?' the pleasant young man asks me as I plonk my backpack down.

'Sharing,' I say.

'Right,' he says. 'And how many nights?'

I tell him two nights. I'm keen to do a more purposeful wander tomorrow when I'm feeling stronger.

'Okay, you're in a six-bedded bunk room. I'd get up there early, if I was you. We're going to be full tonight.'

I decide to take his advice and, thanking him, I drag myself up to the room on the second floor.

Gosh I'm tired, I could sleep for a week.

I open the door and see three bunk beds squashed into a small room. I'm the first one there and so I grab a bottom bed near a window, unpack my sleeping-bag and minutes later I'm asleep.

It feels like I have hardly slept when I'm woken by voices speaking loudly in German. My bleary eyes half-focus on four young men who have walked into the room. They don't see me in the shadows and so one of them throws his backpack onto my bed. A rude awakening. I sit up and peer at the young man whose pack had just nailed me. He's tall and has the long hair and wispy beard that I associate with the flower children of the 60s.

'Sorry, so sorry,' he stammers in heavily accented English when he realises there's a person on the bed. 'I did not see you there.' There's a mix of embarrassment and concern in his voice when he asks, 'Are you all right?'

'I'm fine,' I reassure him. 'Just sleeping. I had a bit of a rough night last night.'

The bag thrower introduces himself as Dieter and then introduces me to his friends. They're political science students from Hamburg. Bound by the commonality of our travelling experiences, we chat amicably. We swap stories about our ferry crossings. It turns out that we'd been on the same ferry. Irritatingly, they'd had a good night. There is much laughter, especially when I tell them about Dylan, Nolan and co.

'So you are from Australia?' Dieter asks.

My accent makes this a common assumption.

'No,' I say.

'New Zealand?' I shake my head. Dieter is puzzled. 'But you don't sound English or American … so where are you from?' he asks, smiling.

'South Africa.'

You could have sworn that I had just ripped off my jacket to expose a bomb. Dieter leaps back from me and talks in rapid angry German to his friends. They all scowl at me. I'm completely nonplussed. What on earth is going on?

'You filthy racist!' Dieter screams at me. 'Get out!'

'What?' I stare at him, bewildered. I don't understand what's happened.

'You heard me – get out!' he shouts. 'We will not sleep in the same room as a fascist racist pig like you!'

'But ... but ...' I protest. 'I'm not a racist.'

'You're South African, you're a racist! And you and your kind disgust me,' Dieter says with a sickening righteousness.

Now I'm getting angry and indignant. 'You don't know anything about me!' I shout back, adrenalin coursing. 'This is ridiculous. It's like me asking you to leave because I hold you responsible for the Holocaust!'

Prejudice defies logic, however, and they're not budging.

'Get out, now!' they say again threateningly.

I've never been much of a fighter, not in the physical sense, that is, so after hesitating just a moment longer, I pick up my things and leave. Still shaking with shock and anger, I go downstairs and explain what has happened to the young man at reception. 'I'm sorry,' he says. 'I could try and talk to them, if you want?'

'No, thanks,' I reply. I'm not going back there.

'Well, there's a single room you can have, but only for one night, and it's going to cost double ...' He's trying to be sympathetic but I feel insult being piled on injury.

I've done nothing to deserve this.

I am being discriminated against, based on nothing more than the accident of my birth.

THE DAYS AFTER Waterford pass in a pleasant blur. I'm entranced by Ireland. I wander, dodging showers and rainbows, from one achingly beautiful Irish landscape to another, experiencing for the first time the joy of being totally free and beholden to no one.

Apart from that first terrible experience, the hostels have been a treat in their own right. Mostly they're old farmhouses some distance from the nearest town but, without fail, warm and welcoming. There are young people from all over the world stopping over in these places and in the evenings groups of us coalesce to cook, play games and go in search of good craic at local pubs. It works like a balm on the memory of my horror of the night in Waterford.

As much as I enjoy company, I also love periods of solitude, so when I read a notice offering a 'quaint 1 roomed cottage, set in isolation in the wilds of the Galway mountains, no electricity, but water from a nearby spring', I don't hesitate. It's 35 km away from where I am and an easy walk. So the notice says.

The following morning I set out, map in hand, along the narrow lane that wends its way up into the surrounding hills. It's a freshly washed, cold, clear morning. The fields, thick with dew, sparkle magically. I feel so alive! The ascent is gentle and as I walk I take pleasure in breathing in the fresh scent of gorse and taking the time to marvel at the tiny blue and yellow flowers that dot the edges of the lane.

A few hours pass. I think that I must have done at least 10 km, so I stop, eat a sandwich and take a long draft from my water bottle. A curious sheep ambles over to the hedge against which I am leaning. They're different to the sheep we have at home; their thick, matted, cream-coloured coats are hung with assorted bits of bramble and heather. She sniffs the air, decides against my sandwich and then ambles away. Apart from a few sheep, I haven't seen another soul and I'm loving it.

I'm making steady progress, or so my map seems to indicate. I'm footsore but very grateful for my new shoes, which I bought on the fly at a bargain store in France. I had only bought one major item for my backpacking adventure, some seriously expensive hiking boots. Two days into my trip the boots hurt so much I had to ditch them on a station platform. I hope they're treating whoever is wearing them now better than they treated me.

I've been walking all day and it begins to dawn on me that I should have reached the cottage by now. I peer through the fast-fading winter light, seeking in vain for any sign of habitation. I can't see a thing, but far from being worried, I feel strangely exultant. I've got everything I need

– a sleeping-bag, food and a waterproof jacket. If necessary, I'll find a sheltering hedge and wait till morning.

I walk on, lost in pleasant thought until, on rounding a bend, I see what must be the cottage, a small stone building tucked into a hollow on the side of the road. It is. A quick look around and I see it's very basic – stone walls and floors, single bed and little else – but it's exactly what I'd hoped for. Tired and happy, I open a tin of baked beans and salvage a bottle of beer from my rucksack. I quickly finish both before collapsing into bed.

I wake with the dawn, which, being winter, is not early. After eating a very stale sandwich, I pack up and consider my next move.

Not for the first, nor the last time in my life, I realise that I've acted impulsively. Shooting first and aiming later. So, typically, I'd not thought beyond getting to this cottage. Looking at the map, it's clear that I have two choices: either walk back the way I've come, or keep going to the next hostel, which is 70 km away. It makes no sense to go back and it's not clear how I'm going to make it to the next hostel, but that's what I decide to do, hoping that in the course of the day, I'll pick up a lift.

It's what the Irish would call a 'soft' day. This is a euphemism for a miserable day – a low grey sky and constant chill drizzle. I'm not fazed, though, and as I stride out I start to sing. I sing all the songs I can remember. Sadly, no one other than the occasional sheep is around to appreciate my repertoire.

I've been walking for at least three hours and I'm no longer feeling so enthused. In fact, I'm feeling pretty miserable. My cheap shoes are letting in water and my feet are cold and wet. My glasses keep fogging up and I'm out of food – my planning could have been better. But the worst is that I haven't seen a car since I started off this morning. Not one. I'm really in the middle of nowhere. Windswept hills covered in gorse and heather roll away in every direction. For a moment, I panic. Flip, I realise, I might have to walk the whole way! After a few deep breaths, a prayer and some motivational self-talk, I calm down and plod on.

Another hour goes by before I think I hear the sound of an approaching car. Or is it just the wind? No – it's a car. Out of the gloom a sleek green Jaguar emerges. I stand in the middle of the road and wave the driver to a stop. There is absolutely no way that I'm going to let him pass!

He rolls down his window. A prosperous-looking middle-aged man, tweed jacket, flat cap. 'Can I help you?' he asks.

'Yes, please,' I say, and then I tell him my story.

'Well, lad,' he says, 'it's your lucky day. I can drop you right at your hostel.' A wave of relief floods over me. 'You put your pack and raincoat in the boot and we'll be off,' he says.

Stuff duly stowed, I climb into his warm, dry car and collapse into the beige leather seat.

'So are you backpacking around Ireland?' he asks, to which I nod, hardly able to speak now that I'm warm and comfortable. He glances as me and smiles. 'And what do you think of it then?'

'It's been great!' I say enthusiastically. 'It's so beautiful and I've found people to be so warm and welcoming.' He smiles again and nods.

After some more small talk and talking (of course) about the weather, I broach a subject that's been on my mind. 'I've been reading the story of Ireland,' I tell him, 'and I was wondering whether it's the long history of oppression that has shaped your people?' He gives a slight frown and throws me another look.

'Possibly ...' he says. 'We've been the underdog for so long that I think we are very mindful to not lord it over others.'

We fall silent for a few minutes. I gaze out of the window at the misty grey and feel grateful all over again that I'm not squelching along on my sore feet.

'So, where are you from then, boyo?' the man asks. And then, before I can answer, and as I have come to expect, he goes through the list: 'Australia?' 'No.' 'New Zealand?' 'No.' And so we continue. 'So where then?' he asks eventually.

'South Africa,' I say.

He glances sideways, frowns and looks away. We settle into what feels to me like a companionable silence interrupted only by the comforting hum of the heater and the swish of the windscreen wipers. My mind wanders … a hot shower … food!

Then, with a sudden stab of his foot, the driver brings both the car and my pleasant reverie to an abrupt halt. I look around. A sheep, a rock perhaps?

'Get out,' he says in a soft voice, looking straight ahead.

'Excuse me?' I say, sure that I've misheard him.

'I said get out,' he says again, louder this time.

'Out of the car? Here?' I say with a smile in my voice. 'Okaay …' I make as if to open the door, waiting for him to confirm the joke. But he makes no move to stop me. 'You can't be serious?' I say in disbelief. 'You want me to get out in the middle of the rain, in the middle of nowhere? Why?'

'I will not share the same space with an oppressor, a black hater,' he snaps.

Perhaps I am better prepared for this because of my encounter with the German students at the Waterford hostel, so this time I shoot back. 'And you know this about me based on what?' I say. 'The colour of my skin?' He hesitates. I continue. Now I am seriously fuming. 'If that's the case, then you're no better than the racists you claim to abhor!'

He reddens. Perhaps he hasn't thought this through but, not willing to back down, he says quietly, 'Just get out.' And so I do.

Having retrieved my pack and coat from the Jag's boot, I stand and watch as its tail-lights recede through the steadily falling rain. I may be cold and wet but my anger warms me. Who does he think he is? How dare he make these assumptions about me? Soon my anger turns into self-pity. Twice this has happened in a week! It's not my fault I'm a white South African. I didn't choose to be born where and what I was.

I wish I could say that I made the connection between the injustice of discrimination that I had just experienced (twice!) and that experienced by millions of South Africans every single day, but I confess I didn't. That insight would only come years later.

By now it's late in the afternoon. I stand dejectedly in the road, the soft Irish rain soaking me all over again in minutes. I am miserable, and feeling extremely sorry for myself. With what I estimate is 20 km to go, I decide there's nothing for it. I have no choice but to plod on. By my rough calculation, if I keep going I should be there by around 9pm. Looking at the rivulets of water on the road, I smile wryly. I may be hungry, but I'm certainly not going to die of thirst. I walk on, still veering between moments of anger and self-pity. Then, just as I'm feeling particularly sorry for myself, I hear the sound of a car approaching. I almost don't dare to hope it will stop, but I wave the old Ford truck down anyway.

The truck comes to a stop. The elderly man, a farmer, I think, beckons me to jump in. Seems like he's not even worried where I'm going. Throwing my pack into the truck-bed, I climb into the cab. We exchange pleasantries and the farmer says he'll take me to the hostel.

And then we get to the dreaded moment.

'So where're you from, lad?' he asks.

'Zimbabwe,' I reply.

'Where's that then?' he asks.

I smile.

6.

JUNGLE DOCTOR

The midday heat is heavy on my back. Despite my hopes for the bronzed look, the best my skin can do is produce a mish-mash of freckles. If I'm lucky, some of them may join forces and give me the tan I'm after.

I've been out behind the backline for ages. Every time I think I'm about to catch a wave, it swoops under me, gives me a momentary lift and then leaves me behind. But this one is different. I actually get it. I'm yanked forward – but where once there was water, there is only air and I'm falling. Far below I see the beach rushing up to meet me, but I am not ready to meet it. I see water and sand. Downside is up and upside is down. Eventually the remnants of the wave let me go and spit me onto the beach.

Dazed and coughing, I drag my gawky frame towards my towel, sand dribbling from parts of my body that sand should never reach.

My surfing attempt sums up how I am feeling right now. Sort of tumbled over and spat out. Three schools in a year, acne, braces, sunburned and a shattered self-esteem.

I flop down under the shade of a beach umbrella and, wiping my hands, I reach for my book.

The roar of the waves and the sounds of laughing children recede as my imagination takes hold … transporting me rapidly into East Africa. The unfolding story immerses me. Soon I'm living in its reality. Against a backdrop of the wildness and beauty of an African storm, a young doctor risks his life. He desperately fords a swollen river, racing to save a mother and her unborn child from certain death. On reaching the remote clinic, he is met by the familiar smell of blood, sweat and fear. Shadowy light illuminates the figure of a woman, little more than a girl, lying on a blood-soaked bed. He knows that the only hope is a caesarean section.

'I have never done anything like this before, but I am willing to try,' the young nurse says, her eyes wide.

'Nor have I,' the doctor responds in a whisper.

They say a short prayer and, using only local anaesthetic, begin.

Concentration, muffled words. Scalpel, white gauze turning red, skin then fat then uterine wall and then at last the half-moon cut exposes the baby's head. Urgently, gently, they manoeuvre the baby into this world. Cord cut, the nurse takes the baby and wraps her in a green sheet while the doctor reverses the earlier process, repairing the damage he has inflicted on the mother's young skin. Moments later a baby's cry …

'GARTH, DID YOU hear me? It's lunch-time. It's time to go home for lunch. Garth!'

My mother's voice drags me back into the real world, a sandy beach in South Africa, not the savannas of East Africa. At the same time as she's pulling at the edge of my consciousness, she's pulling at my beach towel and gathering our things into a basket. She plucks the book out of my hand and shakes the sand from its pages.

'*Jungle Doctor Operates*,' she says. 'I thought you'd read this one already.'

I have read it twice. It's one of my favourites from the series. The sound of the waves and children's laughter gradually bring me back to the present. I am reluctant to leave my fantasy. In my mind, it was me who had saved that girl and delivered her baby. Being the hero felt good. It spoke of a life of significance and purpose, temporarily replacing my constant feeling of failure.

My imagination, honed by years of solitary play, reading and listening to radio dramas, is easily ignited by story. Jungle Doctor is a series of books about a missionary doctor bringing help and healing to those in need in inaccessible places and I can't get enough of them. I feel particularly drawn to the savannas of East Africa.

That teenage kid could not know then how he would hang onto those stories like a drowning man in years to come, but they sparked in me the desire to try to be the person I wanted to be. I wanted to be a courageous hero, fighting against the odds, saving people (and in the process winning fair maids). And I wanted to make my dad proud.

AT THE END of my fifth year of medical school an opportunity arises to spend a month with the medical relief group AMREF, the flying doctors, in Kenya – Jungle Doctor territory. Finally, my life is beginning!

Full of hope, I arrive in Nairobi and make my way to the station and a train trip to Mombasa. What should have been a ten-hour trip takes 24 hours. Every so often, without any warning, the train comes to a random halt and there we sit, for hours, in the baking heat of the East African plains, before eventually shuddering on. My fellow travellers are unperturbed in that uniquely African way that accepts what will be will be. What little food and drink people have is readily shared. Children are passed between strangers, including me; music is played and stories shared.

Impatient as I am at times and hot and frustrated, the journey, I will come to understand, is often as important as the destination.

I climb wearily off the crowded train in Mombasa and negotiate my way through a jostling, colourful kaleidoscope of chickens, children and hundreds of people all seemingly moving in different directions. I need to find a bus that will take me up the coast to my rendezvous with Dr Spoerry, the flying doctor I am to accompany to a clinic on the Somali border. With help, I track down the right bus, a matatu, a vehicle of dubious age and lineage, which is gaudily painted and boasts a roof-rack overflowing with its passengers' multiple goods: huge bundles, tightly wrapped, bags, parcels, bicycles, and even a shackled goat, which is bleating mournfully. Barely discernible under layers of ochre-coloured dust on the side of the matatu is the verse 'Fear not for I am with you'. I'm not sure whether this is there to comfort the passengers or to warn them.

Eight bone-jarring hours later we judder to a halt. This is the second leg of my destination – the small coastal village of Mokowe. Retrieving my backpack, I step sluggishly from the bus. AMREF has been very vague. I was to get myself here and then ask for Dr Spoerry. I look around at the cluster of sun-baked buildings, waves of heat rising off their corrugated-iron roofs. The heavy coastal air stirs occasionally, rustling the scrub bush that surrounds the village.

There is not a soul in sight. I'm not sure what I was expecting – maybe an AMREF sign? A clinic? Even another human being would have been nice. Mild panic sets in. I knock on a door. Nothing. Another one. No response. Eventually a door opens.

'Can I help you?' a slight, elderly man asks as he squints at me.

'Please,' I say, relieved. 'I'm looking for Dr Spoerry.' The man looks at me blankly. 'Dr Spoerry? The doctor who flies a plane?' I say desperately. His face breaks into a smile.

'You mean mamadaktari!' he says quickly. There is what sounds like 'doctor' in there so I say yes. 'The doctor stays across the water in Lamu,' he tells me. Then, when I obviously look somewhat baffled, he adds: 'Do you want to go there?'

'Yes, please,' I say fervently.

'Okay. Wait a little for me and I will row you across.'

The man retreats into his house and I wait. And wait.

Eventually, my ferryman emerges, blinking into the late afternoon sun, and we walk the short distance to where a dilapidated rowing boat is drawn up on the beach.

Lamu is a small island separated from the mainland by a narrow channel. Arab traders first established it as a port in the fourteenth century. After a short crossing, the boat crunches onto the beach, finding space between triangular-sailed dhows resting at anchor and an assortment of old wooden boats lying at random on the shore.

'That's the doctor's house,' my guide says, pointing up at a squat ochre block. Built centuries ago, I doubt it has changed much. Thanking him, I disembark and lug my backpack up to the house. I stand before the wood and iron grilled door, grasp the door-knocker and give it a few hearty whacks.

Almost immediately, the heavy door swings open. 'Yes?' a diminutive white-haired lady says, as much in accusation as in greeting.

Taken aback, I stammer, 'Er … I'm here to see Dr Spoerry. I believe he's expecting me?'

A frown crosses her deeply wrinkled face. 'No, he's not expecting you,' she says.

'He's not?' This can't be happening.

'No … but she is,' she says gruffly without the hint of a smile. 'I'm Dr Spoerry. Come in.'

Busted! In my mind Dr Spoerry, the 'flying doctor' of my imagination, is an athletic, sun-bronzed man oozing competence and purpose. Instead, I'm faced with an irritable weather-beaten woman who must be approaching 80.

She leads me down a cool dark passage to my room. It is starkly furnished with an iron bed, a wash-basin and a mosquito net. It smells of damp. 'We eat dinner in an hour,' she says brusquely. 'And we leave at six tomorrow morning.' What have I got myself into, I wonder?

I'm woken early the following morning by the calls to prayer that ring out from the surrounding mosques. After a quick breakfast, I follow a non-communicative Dr Spoerry, retracing my previous day's trip back to the village. The place still seems largely uninhabited; only a few scrawny chickens brave the chill morning air.

'Wait here,' Dr Spoerry says and she strides away, her over-large khaki shirt flapping behind her.

I don't have to wait long. When she reappears she is accompanied by two middle-aged women in nursing uniforms that look weary from washing. They are carrying a cardboard box. Dr Spoerry signals for me to follow them down a dusty track leading out of the village – to the airfield,

I presume, to meet the pilot. A short walk takes us into a bush clearing. A long, rutted track with the grass cut away on either side is, I think, the runway, because at its head is a single-engine plane, its tail emblazoned with a large red cross. There is no one around.

Dr Spoerry, trailed by the nurses, makes purposefully for the plane. No, I think, panicked. She's the pilot! I will someone else to appear, but in vain.

'Come on then, make yourself useful,' Dr Spoerry says to me. 'Help me swing the plane around.'

I have the same feeling I get when a roller coaster starts its ascent. Scared to death but knowing it's too late to pull out.

The four of us climb into the plane and buckle ourselves in. There is a huge pillow on the pilot's seat, but even with its help, Dr Spoerry battles to see over the dashboard. If I'm to die, I hope it's quick.

An hour's turbulent flight later, I exit the plane, nauseous but alive. The surrounding bush is unlike any bush I've seen before. The vast blue sky above and the ochre of the sand below frames its thick emerald foliage.

Waiting for us are two men in a worse-for-wear Land Rover. Apparently, we have a further two hours' drive until we reach the clinic on the Somali border. The assault rifles the men carry reminds me that we are in a war zone. Excitement overcomes my apprehension. This is the Africa and the medicine I have been dreaming of all these years. I opt to stand in the open back of the vehicle and hang on for a wild ride. The warm wind whips my face – it's glorious!

After miles of emptiness, a small building takes shape on the horizon. 'Is that the clinic?' I ask and the man next to me nods.

Finally!

The clinic is barely standing. Overrun by the surrounding foliage, its peeling walls support a rusted corrugated-iron roof. Seated at a wooden table on the veranda is a tired-looking nurse. She stands wearily to greet us. 'Mamadaktari, I am glad you have arrived,' she says. 'There are many people for you to see.'

'Many' is an understatement. There are at least a hundred people, mainly women and children, waiting patiently in a colourful queue snaking into the surrounding bush.

Dr Spoerry turns to walk back to the Land Rover, jerks her head in my direction and says, 'Well, get on with it then.'

I'm flummoxed. Then I realise she's perfectly serious.

I, a fifth-year medical student, am on my own.

Working with the nurses, I try my best. Dehydrated babies. 'Do we have IV fluids?' 'No.' Malaria. 'Do we have any chloroquine?' 'No.' A septic wound. 'Do we have any penicillin?' 'No.' And so it continues. We have nothing! Nothing except the jumbled contents of the cardboard box, namely, a few swabs, creams, vitamins and aspirin.

I feel helpless and angry as I see one patient after another, knowing the time they have spent walking, then waiting in the heat, in the false expectation that they will be helped. For years, my Jungle Doctor dream has sustained me. Once I get out of medical school, it will all be worth it, I have reassured myself, over and over. Now I am almost there and I'm as disillusioned as hell, my certainties thrown into confusion.

It's possible, of course, that my story might have turned out differently if, that day, instead of Dr Spoerry, I had accompanied one of the many real 'flying doctors' who worked then – and still do today – selflessly and professionally to bring medical help and hope to people in remote locations who have limited access to health care.

Crestfallen, I retrace my travels. Land Rover then plane. This time I fly with Dr Spoerry, with a brief stop to drop off the nurses, all the way back to Nairobi.

I try to find out from her whether the clinic I have just been to is an anomaly, possibly a logistics failure. From her gruff, monosyllabic answers, it seems not. She's surprised at my discomfort and I'm surprised at her lack of it. It stays with me for a long time.

Many years later her lack of empathy finally make sense when I come upon a book, *In Full Flight: A Story of Africa and Atonement*, and discover that it is Dr Spoerry's story. A Frenchwoman with questionable medical qualifications, and wanted for war crimes, 'Mamadaktari' had fled Europe to reinvent herself in Africa. During the Second World War, she had been interned in a concentration camp and had collaborated with the Germans in some horrific medical experiments.

The few days I have in Nairobi before flying back home gives me ample time to brood. The reality begins to dawn on me that imagining a story might not be the same as living it. The anxiety this provokes in me is tangible. I want to fast forward the next two years I have before qualifying, to see how this turns out. Maybe what I've just experienced really is an anomaly and the reality is more Paul White, my Jungle Doctor icon, than it is Anne Spoerry. Only time would tell.

THE FLAME OF hope that I might yet be a hero jungle doctor apparently did not completely die out in Kenya. It flared briefly, and unexpectedly, some years later in another lush part of Africa – the densely subtropical KwaZulu-Natal bush.

The circumstances and setting couldn't have been more different, however.

I was with Soul City colleague Harriet Perlman, not in a small, single-engined plane but in a car that was taking some strain on a steep and rocky incline in sweltering heat. Our destination was not a rickety clinic in the middle of nowhere but a luxury lodge with spectacular scenery. Unfortunately, we are not on holiday – we are here to work, hopefully to secure some funding for our cause.

We see a collection of thatched stone buildings that blend into the scenery and a sign that tells us we have come to the right place: Phinda Mountain Lodge.

I'm excited and despite the afternoon heat that comes in debilitating waves, I have a delicious shiver of anticipation.

'You're looking forward to this, aren't you?' Harriet says.

'Sure – aren't you?' I say. 'Did you read the reviews of this place?'

'No,' she says, holding onto the dashboard as we lurch and almost stall.

'Stuff like "spellbinding views", "top end luxury safari", "an experience of a lifetime". And we get to stay for free.'

'You're such an NGO type, Garth,' she laughs.

Harriet is one of Soul City's senior managers and she and I have known each other for years. While she may be short in stature, she is not in aptitude. She is one of the most capable people I know. We are here because we work in this community and we are being showcased at Ted Turner's United Nations Foundation, which is having a board meeting at Phinda.

'It's not just the freebee. It's the opportunity of meeting with Ted Turner, Jane Fonda and their rich board members,' I point out. 'I googled them and they're all billionaires.'

'Well, I feel like a goldfish in a bowl. Rich American do-gooders. See what these nice Africans are doing,' says Harriet. Before she can vent more steam, we crest the rise and come to a dusty standstill at the base of the stone steps leading to the lodge entrance. As we pull up, the large wooden door swings open and a harried-looking middle-aged man in bush khaki rushes down the steps towards us.

'You're a doctor, aren't you?' he says. No preamble. No welcome.

'Yes,' I reply, confused.

'Come quickly, please! One of Mr Turner's guests ate some peanuts and now he can't breathe,' he says desperately.

I haven't practised clinically for a while, but I remember that a peanut allergy can quickly be life-threatening. A real medical emergency. Without adrenalin, there is only one option: an emergency tracheotomy. Making an incision just below the Adam's apple and them ramming some sort of tube in to bypass the obstruction. I've read about it but never done it.

'Take me to your kitchen!' I say in my most authoritative, I've-got-this-under-control voice, while Harriet looks bemused.

'The kitchen?' the man says.

'Yes. I need a sharp knife and a straw,' I say. 'Hurry!'

We take the steps two at a time and I follow him down a passage and into a busy kitchen. 'This man needs a sharp knife – now!' the lodge manager says to a startled chef. He can see from our wild expressions that this is not the time for questions and presents us with an array of lethal-looking knives.

'That one,' I say, pointing to a particularly wicked small blade. 'And I'll need a straw.' A paper drinking straw is quickly found and placed into my other hand.

The manager and I rush out of the kitchen and through the lodge, me brandishing the knife and straw, bouncing amazed guests and staff out of our way. I'm sure we are quite a sight.

We arrive in the sitting room. Ground zero. My adrenalin surges. There is nothing like the thought of slitting a man's throat while he's awake to sharpen the senses.

Except there is no one there.

'They've taken him to the airstrip,' one of the waiters says.

Turning urgently, the manger beckons me to follow him. 'We'll try and catch them,' he says.

Moments later, we are lurching at breakneck speed though the bush. I cling tightly onto the bucking Land Rover. Maybe I'll die before we reach the patient. The prospect of 'jungle doctor' bush surgery is rapidly losing its appeal. We emerge through the trees just in time to see a plane hurtle down the runway and lift into the air, destination Richards Bay hospital.

The Land Rover comes to an abrupt halt. I'm covered in sweat. I look down at my shaking hands, knife in the one and straw in the other.

A straw! What the – It hits me. Cold relief washes over me. A straw! If I had cut through the man's cricothyroid membrane and into his trachea and then threaded the straw through for an airway, as I had been intending to do, the negative pressure would have collapsed the straw and the man would surely have died. I shudder, visualising the headlines: 'Doctor Murders American Billionaire at Exclusive Game Lodge'. Not a great fund-raising tactic.

Bloody idiot. How could I be so dumb? A fresh wave of sweat breaks over me. I needed a *pen* not a *straw*. You take the ink cartridge out and use the stiff tube to insert. No airway collapse and no dead person.

Arriving back at the lodge, I recount my close shave to Harriet.

'His close shave,' she corrects me. 'Do you really think you could have killed him?' She is quite astonished.

I nod weakly. 'I just can't believe how lucky I was. A few minutes earlier and ...' I make a slitting gesture across my throat.

Harriet suddenly starts laughing.

'What's funny?' I ask irritably.

'You know the saying "the pen is mightier than the sword"?'

'Ja ...'

'Well, in your case it should be "the pen is mightier than the straw"!'

She thinks this is hilarious. I don't, I'm still in shock. I almost killed a man.

7.

DARK CITY, SOUL CITY

I always hear the children's clinic before I see it. A multitude of wails and whimpers. Who would have thought that such tiny beings could make such noise? Actually, I have learned to welcome the sound. It's when a child is silent that you should really worry. Thankfully, no silent kids today, but it's been a long one, with the queue miraculously refilling whenever I think we are done.

Finally, and to my relief, Sister Theresa smiles and signals to me, 'last one', as she leads a young mother and child to my cubicle.

Some people shape you without knowing it. Sister Theresa shaped me. A small, upright woman in her early 60s, glasses fighting a losing battle with gravity on her nose, for the last 20 years she has run the paediatric unit at Alexandra Clinic. In that time she has seen many young doctors come and go and yet, even though she knows so much more than me, she has guided and often forgives me as I attempt to run the unit.

I lean forward and, in my halting Zulu, enquire about the child. But I already know what's wrong. Sunken eyes, dry mouth and where there should be a full fontanelle a black-coated depression. Yet another child dehydrated from vomiting and diarrhoea.

'How long has the child been sick, Ma?'

The child's mother looks at me, surprised and definitely confused.

Apparently my Zulu is not as good as I think it is, but before I can wonder what it is I have actually said, Sister Theresa quickly intervenes.

It's the same story. I have heard it every day for the last two years.

The vomiting and diarrhoea is attributed to a bad spirit, 'Injoni'. The treatment? Sister Theresa has taught me well and I recognise the mother's best efforts – a black substance pasted onto the fontanelle, to prevent more bad spirits getting into the body, and enemas to flush them out. I've learned that sometimes cultural practices are helpful but not in these cases; this treatment just makes matters worse.

While the child will need a drip to rapidly rehydrate him, he should be fine. Unlike the three children who arrived dead at the clinic this week. It breaks my heart that something so preventable should still be the leading cause of death of children under the age of five. No child should ever die of dehydration.

With her usual patience and compassion, Sister Theresa talks to the mother, pointing at the huge colourful mural on the unit's wall depicting the life-saving salt, water and sugar solution that can be administered at home.

I am always looking for innovative ways to communicate with patients and getting this mural painted was one of my better ideas. Much better than the huge hydrogen balloon I hired to float over the clinic with the words 'Come and vaccinate your child today!' on it. Kids flocked to the clinic ... but to see the balloon, not to be vaccinated! The tea room was never the same after that.

'Hey, Garth, how's the balloon?'

'Always thought you were full of hot air ...'

Sister Theresa is talking to me. 'Doctor, are you on casualty tonight?' she asks. 'You can take the child with you, if you are.'

Suddenly I'm whacked in the gut.

I am. I am on casualty tonight.

I feel my shoulders tighten. My anxiety, always lurking, instantly makes its presence felt. While the paediatric clinic is busy, it's not wild. Casualty is wild. I have only been out of med school three years and, as Sister Theresa has just reminded me, tonight I will be 'it', along with the nursing staff and two sixth-year medical students.

This casualty is the primary medical facility for Alexandra township. For the many years it went without electricity, which left the township pitch-dark at night, and Alex earned its nickname – 'Dark City'. But my experience is that Alex is anything but dark. Rather it is a vibrant, colourful, ever-changing community, full of life, despite oppression and trouble.

Walk down any dusty street and you will pass sturdy old 'four rooms' cheek by jowl with an amazing variety of lean-to structures, a testament to human ingenuity. People are everywhere, dodging hooting taxis, shouting greetings to one another and scolding the children who make the streets their playgrounds. Gogos who have spent their whole lives in Alex mix seamlessly with the endless flow of new arrivals from every part of the country and continent. Some are full of hope and swagger; others are disorientated, far from their pastoral homes.

No matter what time of the day, music cascades through open doors, washing over men as they nurse their quarts. The smell of coal smoke, raw sewage and rubbish mixes with the allure of pap and steak grilling on open fires. So alluring, in fact, that I would often drive around looking for my weekly fix, that was, until I got mugged for my trouble.

Things happen fast in Alex. In an instant, laughter can turn to tears and peace to terror.

IT'S 1992 – PRE-DEMOCRACY – and there has been a steady escalation of violence as the ANC and Inkatha jockey for position.

It's worst at night as men go to war – pangas, petrol bombs, guns and knives – in fact, anything that can kill or maim and God help you if you get in the way.

Sometimes my anxiety is misplaced. Not tonight.

I walk into casualty. Things are quiet. Swing doors open from the street into a well-ordered space permeated by the smell of surgical spirits, which tries valiantly to mask the smell of old blood. Ten beds in all. The monotony of the floor-to-ceiling linoleum is broken up by the variety of paraphernalia that make up a casualty unit. Sterile surgical packs mummified in green, trays of needles, syringes and bottles of disinfectant. Drip tubing, IV solutions, scalpels, suture material and oxygen cylinders complete the picture.

I wonder who the sister in charge is tonight. I hope it's Anna Mokoena – and it is.

Built broad, powerful and low to the ground, Sister Anna always puts me in mind of a rhino. You don't want to mess with her … that is, until she smiles. Not many people can frighten a raging man full of drink and blood, but Sister Anna can. Standing her ground firmly, I have seen her wave her formidable fists in such men's faces. 'You can choose which one! This one will send you to the mortuary and this one to ICU!'

Sister Anna greets me with her irresistible smile and I smile in return. 'I have a feeling we will be quiet tonight, doctor,' she says.

'From your lips to God's ears, sister.' I look around. 'Have we got students tonight or is it just us?'

Just then two medical students walk in. A young man not shaving yet and a woman who appears to have got out of school early. I'm 28 and I feel old in comparison.

I've been doing a weekly night shift for the last two years and when I am able to shelve the terror of the unexpected, I find it exhilarating. Mostly it's so practical, you can really help the astonishing array of young and old that call Alex home. Dehydrated babies, children with broken limbs and asthma attacks, and the variety of souls that either walk or are carried in with cuts, stabs and gunshot wounds – gifts from Alex.

I mentioned it was quiet tonight. It's too quiet.

It's 8pm and so far we have only seen a toddler with a high temperature. We sit chatting, snacking on the standard medical fodder of chips and Coke, waiting. Nine o'clock comes and goes. Still no one.

And then it happens. A volley of single shots. We duck. It feels like the gunmen are just outside the door. Then the regular pop-pop escalates into a barrage of sound as if a maniac has been let loose on the drums. I peer out of the window that looks onto the adjacent street. I see people running, their bodies shadowed and lit amber by the shacks that have just been set alight.

The doors burst open. Two young men drag their comrade in. His entry is marked by red splashes on the once-clean floor.

'Help him! Now! He has been shot.'

Habit and adrenalin kick in. Sister Anna and I get the man onto the closest bed. She reaches for a pair of scissors and scythes through his designer jacket. 'Stop!' shouts one of his friends. 'That's his best jacket!'

'You want us to help him? Then get out of the way.' Sister Anna doesn't even have to bare her fists. They back off at her tone and the look she gives them. 'Mfuwethu – what is your name?'

The young man is pale and unresponsive. His blood pressure is unrecordable and his breathing ragged. He has a single gunshot wound to the chest, a dark hole from hell oozing blood. It always amazes me how some people walk into casualty red-slicked and body in tatters, looking like they have fought off a pride of lions and survived, but a single stab wound or a bullet in the right place can mean death.

The bullet has lodged in his lung, destroying vessels in its path, and while he may not appear to be bleeding much, his chest is rapidly filling up with blood, constricting his heart and lungs in the process.

Before I have to ask, Sister Anna is already unwrapping the chest drain pack. The two students hover, the young man looking pale. I feel sympathy. Right through med school, I often fainted at the sight of blood.

'Put up a drip while I work,' I tell the student. Keeping him busy will help.

Putting in a chest drain in a hurry is not delicate, but it is life saving. By relieving the pressure, it makes it possible for the heart and lungs to function again. I cut through the muscle between the ribs and then stick a metal spike carrying a tube into the chest cavity. Seconds later dark blood pours into the waiting bottle. Breathing eases and blood pressure rises. He should be okay.

But this is just the beginning. The sounds of war continue unabated and soon one casualty becomes 50. Men, women and children, some dead and some close to death. Gunshot wounds, burns and stab wounds. Will I ever forget the young girl hacked in the chest, her lung exposed? How, oh Lord, can human beings do this to each other, let alone this poor child? I believe in evil as well as good, but sometimes it's easier to believe in evil.

Soon we are overwhelmed.

'Where are the ambulances, sister?' I ask tersely. We can stabilise patients, but most of them need to get to a proper hospital urgently.

'They won't come,' Sister Anna says. 'They say it is too dangerous.'

'The police?'

'Same story. They won't come either, and nor will the army. They say they will come in the morning.'

I am gobsmacked. 'So we are on our own?'

A nod. We get back to work.

The next few hours take me to the brink. We do what we can, but that's often not much. And then there is my background fear. Only a week back, some thugs had invaded the clinic and tried to finish off a guy before we could save him. Were we about to be invaded again? The sound of glass shattering sends us all to the floor. I look up to see a neat hole in one of the windows. I am scared. Am I a man with too much imagination and too little physical courage? I fear I may be.

Sister Anna summons me. 'Please come and see this young man, I need your opinion.'

Lying on a bed, eyes closed and not moving, is a young man in his 20s. He looks peaceful, no sign of any injury. Then Sister Anna lifts up his head, revealing a sticky mess of dark matted hair. Gunshot wound to the back of his head. Entry, no exit. His pulse, blood pressure and breathing reasonable.

A few years earlier I had done neurology at Baragwanath Hospital so I was pretty good at assessing brain function or the lack of it. In his case it was lack of it. He was alive because of his brainstem, the reptilian part of our brain that keeps us alive, but it was clear that he had massive damage to all his higher functions. If he lived, he would most likely neither walk nor talk again. In the midst of the chaos I make a snap decision. 'Leave him be.'

IT'S 3AM. THINGS have quietened down. There are bodies everywhere, but no new casualties. I have sent the medical students to bed and I am now desperate for rest. I retire to the small doctor's room and collapse. I can't sleep as the sounds of automatic rifle fire continue to invade my skull. I'm a wreck. How on earth do people survive a war? I know I couldn't.

At 6am, as I am preparing to go back to casualty, I get a call from a local radio station, although how they got my number is a mystery. Already the news is full of last night's happenings in Alex and they want to hear direct from me. I'm struck by how different it feels to be *in* the horror story that is the news rather than just being one of the observers morbidly fascinated by the statistics of death and suffering. Years later in the time of COVID-19 this experience will give me insights into the sense of isolation felt by many health-care workers dealing daily with fatigue, unimaginable choices, and the trauma experienced by both patients and families. They leave their hospitals into what feels like a foreign land of recipe swapping and statistics.

I will learn that that night, 60 people were killed in Alex, nearly 600 people were injured and around 10 000 people were displaced from their homes.

Finally I make it back to casualty. It's astonishing how daylight can transform a scene. There are a queue of ambulances outside and Sister Anna is making sure that the most urgent patients get taken first. She gives me a smile. 'I told you it would be a quiet night.' I can only grimace in reply.

'Let's start the handover,' I say.

Waiting for us is a distinguished-looking doctor, neatly clipped moustache, a smattering of grey fringing his hair. He is the clinic's medical manager and a recent returnee from exile. He is both invigorated and appalled at the birth pangs of the 'new' South Africa. 'Rough night?' he asks.

We go through each patient: what's the diagnosis and what's the plan? Medical students and nursing staff are in tow. Then we get to the young man. The man with a bullet in his brain. Still alive.

'Why has he no drip or even oxygen?' the medical manager asks, and I explain my reasoning.

What happens next blindsides me. The man explodes. 'I am certain that if he were white you would not have treated him like this!' he says. 'What gives you the right to decide? Who do you think you are?'

And so it continues. I do not know what to say. My denials sound like admissions of guilt.

Last night had shattered me but this shatters me in a different way.

I think I am here in Alex because I care. I want to use my privilege for good and this man, a man I respect, is calling this into question. Is he right?

As I drive home, shock begins to turn to indignation. He made a judgement call about me based on my appearance. Not only does he not know my story, he doesn't even know the full story from last night. What would he have done in the same circumstances?

But can I blame him? I am equally guilty of judging people based on what I think I know about them, often merely based on their appearance. Do I know *his* story? Maybe, not, I am sure that if we had taken the time to find out each other's stories, our conversation would have been a whole lot different. Perhaps, instead of anger and frustration and resentment on both sides, the picture would have looked more like this: an experienced doctor supporting an inexperienced one at the end of a harrowing night.

Again and again, my journey through life will show me how knowing someone's personal story can make a world of difference in how we react or respond, in words, and actions, and behaviour. Of course we do not all have the time – nor take the time – to understand one another, and circumstances and situations change. One constant, however, is that storytelling, in whatever format, remains one of the most powerful vehicles for transformation. Often the most effective way of getting a point across is to illustrate it in story form for a receptive audience.

Dark City was the inspiration for what would become the storytelling drama series Soul City.

Radio and television were the platforms.

A CAR DOOR slams. It's a sound that always heralds action. Senses sharpen. Anxiety and anticipation compete as the casualty staff wait for the clinic doors to burst open. They do. The clatter of running feet is drowned out by a mother's hysteria and a child's cries. A distraught mother, clutching her blanket-wrapped child, is followed closely by an older woman who is desperately trying to pull her back to the car.

'Yoh, whe ma, he's been burned, he's been burned!' the mother cries.

It's pandemonium. Both women are screaming as the security guard wrenches the old lady away.

'They'll kill him here!' she cries.

A nurse moves rapidly from behind the counter and takes the child from the mother. 'What happened, Ma?' she says, removing the blanket. There are only sobs in response. She turns to the old woman. 'Gogo, tell us how the child was burned?' The gogo is not much better, but the basic facts of a familiar story emerge. The two-year-old boy was playing in their shack when his mother went outside. A pot of porridge had been left on the stove. The mother, hearing a scream, had rushed inside to find that the child had grabbed the pot handle, sending a cascade of scalding porridge over his body.

'Valeron drops stat!' the doctor barks. The child wails and writhes in agony. 'What a complete mess!' There is exasperation in his voice. Sheets of dark skin hang in ragged clumps from the child's chest, exposing patches of pink flesh. 'Is this what I think it is, sister?' The doctor points to islands of dark paste, partially obscuring the burn. The sister nods. 'Why don't these people ever learn?' he exclaims.

The nurse, a woman not easily intimated, responds. '"These people", as you put it, doctor, are doing the very best they know how by applying shoe polish to the burn. The gogo is convinced she's done the right thing and that bringing the child here is a death sentence.'

'Okay, okay, I get it. It's just so bloody frustrating,' he responds.

'Well, be thankful it's just polish,' the sister says quietly as she tries to soothe the child. 'Cow dung is often used.' The child whimpers as his terrified mother and granny look on.

'Dammit, sister! The emergency treatment for a burn is water, the colder, the quicker.'

'I know that, doctor,' she placates him.

'Ja, but clearly they don't. Polish, dung ... I just don't get it.' He pauses as he reaches for his stethoscope. 'How on earth are we going to get this across to them?'

'Not by shouting,' the sister replies, a sardonic smile on her lips.

The doctor leans over to listen to the toddler's chest.

Oh blast!

I signal frantically to Bobby, the director.

The doctor has the stethoscope back to front.

'Cut! Cut!' the director roars as he emerges from behind his monitor. 'What's the problem, Garth?'

I explain and proceed to show the actor how to use the stethoscope. My seven years of medical training is finally vindicated!

The setting is authentic – we are in Alexandra Clinic – but the scene, while familiar and no less authentic, is dramatised. The participants are actors and crew. We are filming the first episode of the TV drama series we initially called Dark City. But that title sounded a little 'dark', we decided, and lacking 'soul', so Soul City it became.

Understanding my story has been healing for me; now I'm trying to tell stories to heal others, which is a story in itself!

The cries of waiting children and the murmur of their care givers are overshadowed by an unfamiliar mechanical hum. A casual observer would see 'patients' but a closer look would reveal not one cough or temperature among them. The usually spotless linoleum floors are cluttered with cables, steel boxes and light stands. Art is imitating life.

In the middle of the room, a bank of globes forms an island of light in which the scene is being played out. Giant shadows dance on the walls mirroring the action. At the perimeter of the light, the sound guy, his bullet head bracketed by headphones, holds a rod from which protrudes a furry oblong object. To my eyes it looks like he's skewered a cat.

The temporary pause in the filming has unleashed a flurry of movement. The make-up lady dashes in to apply powder to sweaty faces; the sound guy rapidly adjusts knobs and dials; the cameraman fiddles with his camera.

'So Garth, how are you enjoying the shoot so far?' Bobby enquires.

'It's a complete mind blow, it all feels so real!' I say, realising how the burn scene has sucked me in and set my pulse racing.

Bobby Heaney is one of the country's leading directors. A slight, bespectacled man, he seems to be in perpetual motion. What's infectious is how enthused he is with the potential to use his craft to educate while entertaining.

'Did you ever imagine this day would arrive?' he asks.

'No,' I answer truthfully. 'It does feel pretty miraculous.'

This last week has tested my faith and resolve to the limit. There have been times when it looked like we were going to have to abandon the filming. I feel sick just thinking about it, about all we've been through.

We're filming in the war zone that is Alexandra township right now. It's 1993 and isolated sparks of political violence are being fanned by a 'third force' hell-bent on derailing the national peace talks that are currently under way.

Every day I meet with community leaders and every day the response is the same: 'It's too dangerous. We can't guarantee your safety.' And then yesterday, for reasons that I still can't fathom, the answer is 'Yes – go ahead!'

Bobby nods. 'Agreed, Garth. It does feel like this is meant to happen.'

And I do feel that it is meant to. I am strangely comforted. Surely God has not brought us this far only for this project to be birthed into a country at war?

Bobby moves back to his monitor. 'Bobby,' I call after him. 'I've got one request.'

'And what might that be?' he asks cautiously.

'Can you use the word "filming" instead of "shooting"? It feels more appropriate given the circumstances.'

He chuckles before turning to his assistant director. 'Let's get *filming!*' he shouts.

'Quiet, please,' the assistant director orders. 'And … action!'

The doctor bends over the badly burned child and, using the stethoscope like a seasoned pro, listens to his chest.

IN OTHERS' WORDS ...

Some of my happiest times as a child were when my mother read to me, which she did a lot. The rhythm and lilt of another's voice as a story unfolds is a powerful signal to the listener's imagination. I also loved listening to radio dramas, often pretending to be sick so that I could stay home from school to listen to the morning serials. The little blue portable radio I had been given as a gift was a gift indeed. In the evening there were other programmes that held me captive: *Squad Cars*, *The Men From the Ministry*, *Taxi*, *The Mind of Tracy Dark* ... each offering its own special drama, thrill, mysterious crime to be solved, psychological twists and turns, and, of course, comedy. I entered these worlds willingly and the stories I absorbed every day became an integral part of mine.

Ivan Moroke's mother was a strong influence in encouraging him to read. They struggled financially but she made sure there was material in the house to read. 'I grew up on *Reader's Digest*,' Ivan laughed when I asked him about this. 'If there is one thing that shaped my mind it has been *Reader's Digest*. That is what I got from her. The interest or appetite for reading.'

Sometimes we come to our own stories through reading or hearing those of others. A story might resonate with us emotionally on a deep level so that we feel connected and affirmed. A story can illuminate – a time, a place, a period in history – from different angles, to challenge our preconceptions and assumptions. A story can comfort and transport when you are in a lonely space.

'A book is the branch you hold onto when the river sweeps you away,' is how Gcina Mhlophe described her relationship with reading to me. Stories were an integral part of her world, first the ones her grandmother told to her and later, when she learned to read, the stories in books. Her grandmother, with whom she lived in Hammarsdale in KwaZulu-Natal, was a master storyteller and a loving and lively presence in her life. Moving from the green rolling hills of KwaZulu-Natal to Mount Frere in the Eastern Cape, where she attended school, far away from everything and everyone she had known, came as a shock to young Gcina. She chose to excel in her studies and she devoured the written word. Books became a source of comfort, knowledge and wonder – and she also fell in love with the Xhosa language. She discovered AC Jordan and SEK Mqhayi, the latter known as 'the father of Xhosa poetry', and she developed a passionate love of language. Later, after she had finished school, she continued to read voraciously – Es'kia Mphahlele, Sol Plaatje, Miriam Tlali, Mariama Bâ, Cyprian Ekwensi, Chinua Achebe, Efua Sutherland. 'It was like being re-educated, reading my people,' she says.

Gcina's distinctive, expressive voice lent itself to the spoken word, to radio storytelling, to performance poetry and group storytelling. Her audiences, big and small, over the many years she has practised and perfected her craft, continue to be moved by her. 'Story is the mother of all art forms,' she said. 'It allows for intergenerational communication, and it can take many different forms.' She laughed, the sound infectious. 'See what a person can do when you are in full flight with praise poetry!'

In my interview with Laura Dison from Wits, she described some of the interesting work around writing and framing story that she and colleagues conduct at post-grad level with Education students. 'There's a very strong emphasis in academic writing on voice, argument, position and where you stand when it comes to particular claims. Students really struggle with that. Students often think that having their own voice means having an opinion and in some cases their own theory. So we work a lot with the students to develop the confidence and proficiency to ask the questions and critically discuss something and be able to engage with it in a way that shows they thought about it. Students often start telling before they show. Before they have the information, before they have the details, before they have the knowledge.' By introducing a writing method to demonstrating the power of storytelling, students were better able to embrace the richness of description.

Olefile Masangane had his eyes opened and horizons broadened by many of the books he read in his youth. He learned about Botswana through Bessie Head, Kenya through Ngũgĩ wa Thiong'o, Nigeria through Chinua Achebe, and Swaziland through Senzenjani Lukhele. These writers and their creative imaginations inspired him to want to travel and explore other places and cultures for himself, something he came to do through joining Youth for Christ when he was still in high school. But it was a book that a pastor walked him through after sensing an internal struggle during team sessions, that had caused him to walk out, lose interest and not fully participate, that allowed something to shift. The book was called *Twelve Steps to Freedom* and along with it, triggered by a particular song that was regularly sung in church, a difficult memory surfaced. At around 12 years old Ole had been molested by a paedophile and he had never talked about it to a soul. Healing came from going back and confronting that part of his story, Olefile says, but sharing it was his gift. 'It is no longer my story now. It belongs in the world. It belongs to every young boy …'

I came across Alison Harris by chance. This extraordinary young woman was a guest speaker at my children's school and they were moved by a particular story she told about a homeless man in her community of Woodstock, known only as Gary, and how his generous and loving spirit had enriched many lives. She acknowledges Gary and his story as foundational not only in her personal growth but also in realising that she wanted to connect with people, children especially, and make a positive impact on their lives and empower them to realise their dreams. The outreach programmes and organisations she went on to develop, such as the innovative Sk8 for Gr8, which pairs designers, kids and skateboards, are testament to her passion and integrity.

Like most of us, Alison did not find it easy to confront and own aspects of her story, but she found the value of sharing in a safe space. Her first experience of this was during a social entrepreneurship workshop with her peers. 'We all started telling our story and I shared. There was a time in my life when my parents struggled with money. I have no idea how my parents afforded a private high school, it does not make sense. There were times when money was incredibly tight. Telling them about my education and that I still have a student loan and I am still paying that off, so many people were shocked by that. And the one woman actually stood up and said, "I did not know that white people struggle." Everyone in that group had their education paid for and assumed the same of me. I could have gone to the victim mentality but it was such a powerful moment. In the same breath, through listening I also realised that privilege isn't simply monetary. Through listening to each other, we all connected on a deeper level of understanding each other's story and breaking racial stigmas. Realised that we are all human and we all go through stuff. It created a space that was quite beautiful where we all connected on a human level and everything else, in that moment, kind of fell away. That for me made me start a journey and understand and find my own identity in that.'

Her experience of Gary, the homeless man in his 60s, who, for some time, took up residence on her stoep, also brought home to her how easy it is to profile someone when you really know nothing about them.

'Gary would beg for particular food. It would be the chakalaka with extra spice; Koo baked beans and not any other brand. The neighbourhood got to know these very specific things and it became a joke. We would ask him why and he would just say, "No, I want that food." If we did not have that food, he would very politely say, "No, thank you."' Gary had clearly had a hard life, some of which he shared with Alison, and he struggled with alcoholism. The two formed a bond of friendship and after Gary died Alison posted on Facebook the time and date of the memorial service her church organised in Woodstock. The hall was packed. 'People from different walks of life, religion, races – all started to share about Gary. The most impactful story was when a Muslim lady walked up to the front and she told us the reason behind these specific canned foods. Her family had been going through huge financial turmoil, and within her family there is a lot of shame around that. The only person that she could tell was Gary. He knew them like he knew all of us. He really took time to know us and he knew their specific dietary requirements. All this time he was begging for food for her family and he never told us because he knew the shame behind it. He did it without payment or anything and it was just out of his heart. That story inspired me not to judge a book by its cover even when you think you know it.'

It was Alan Paton's *Cry, the Beloved Country* that made a lasting impact on Michael Charton and got him thinking about South Africa's story and how it was being told. As a privileged white South African boy, a chartered accountant with a career comfortably mapped out for him, he had never paid much attention to his fellow countrymen and the history that had shaped them. But absorbing history by reading as widely as he could remained in a sense one-dimensional for him. In sharing his growing passion for history, he began talking to small groups of people, friends and friends of friends at first, and then broadening that audience as people became engaged in the way he told a story. Michael saw how the light goes on inside a person when you tell a story that shows their common humanity, how through story we engage on a fundamental human level. What if he could find an even more imaginative way to tell the rich and multi-faceted stories of our country's past? It was out of this thinking and a memorable experience at Rorke's Drift with historian and storyteller David Rattray that his storytelling show *My Father's Coat* evolved. Retelling the stories of historical heroes and anti-heroes – Shaka, Kruger, Rhodes – but allowing his audience first to meet them individually as children, with all the human emotions – fear, joy, pain – common to us all, he discovered, was a powerful entry point. 'If you know more about people, you have a different take on them,' Michael said during our interview, 'even if they're very different to you. At the very least, you can make people think.'

Heroic characters and why we are so drawn to them is an aspect of story that has always held a fascination for me and I am not alone in this.

At the forefront of scientific work being done internationally on uncovering some of the reason why story is so compelling is Paul Zak, a professor of economics, psychology and management at Claremont Graduate University in the United States. He analysed the types of stories that worked and found that most of them followed the narrative structure of the 'hero's journey', the term that was made famous by the writer Joseph Campbell in his 1949 book *The Hero with a Thousand Faces*. A character goes on a journey, comes up against trials and tribulations and triumphs, despite the odds, ending the journey changed.

I first met Buhle Dlamini when he was working for the Salvation Army as their youth mobiliser. I recognised something extraordinary in him. I said to him that if ever he left the Salvation Army please would he let me know. He did and soon afterwards came to join Heartlines as its third employee. A gifted and natural storyteller, who is now much in demand as an international speaker, Buhle used drama in his international Youth for Christ storytelling platform. Whilst Michael Charton used important figures in our country's history from previous centuries to inspire and intrigue, Buhle chose the dramatic retelling of the stories of more recent heroes, such as Steve Biko, and drew parallels with countries such as Rwanda and Germany. At the same time as South Africans were celebrating democracy in 1994 as a result of the courage and determination of many who strove for a different shape for the country, another country on the African continent, Rwanda, was experiencing the pain and devastation of genocide. In dramatising a character living through that devastating time, Buhle shone a vibrantly honest and deeply moving light on what was happening there. Through humanising two different historical narratives, a deeper understanding is reached.

Cartoonist Jonathan Shapiro (Zapiro) can frame a whole story with depth and provocation in a single frame. His contribution to making South Africans think about who they are and how they behave – located within the current political context – has a powerful impact. 'Everything I do is built around story,' he told me. His mother, whose Jewish roots were in Germany, was his storyteller influence. When he was a young boy, he was drawn to the Giles cartoon compilations; even though he might not have understood their social and political commentary, he found the method, 'sitcom cartooning', compelling. 'A cartoon can capture a moment of history', he said. It challenges people to 'join the dots', think about something in a different way; it allows them to be part of the discourse. 'Once you've seen it, you cannot unsee it.'

This was true for Pastor Leigh Robinson. When he was 18 years old, this traditional white South African travelled to Canada to do training for ministry. Whilst doing outreach ministry one Sunday, going door to door with the hope of sharing the gospel, a woman recognised his accent and invited him inside. She showed him a book called *House of Bondage*, a compilation of photographs by South African photographer Ernest Cole. The images showed the stark reality of life under apartheid South Africa, a side of his country's story he had never even come close to seeing. The stories these evocative and haunting photographs told has never left him.

Actor David Dennis, currently head of the School of Live Performance at AFDA film school, knows more than most about the long-reaching effect and responsibility that comes with playing a memorable, relatable character called Sol in the 1990s' television series Soul City. In our interview I asked him why he believed the impact of story is so profound. 'I think it is to do with our oral tradition,' he said. 'Children love stories. That inner child in all of us will never lose that mystery of the unfolding word as it comes to you. As the storyteller gives it to you. Chooses the image they want to plant in your imagination. It allows ownership of the story to the listener. Ownership in the sense of partnership in the story, in receiving the story.'

Universal stories with an underlying message of honour, integrity, justice and the consequence of one's actions have always resonated with both Seth Naicker and Anele Nzimande. For Seth, the 'pound of flesh' exchange and theme of justice that is central to Shakespeare's *The Merchant of Venice*, which he had as a school setwork, has stayed with him. Similarly, the Grimms fairy tale 'The Pied Piper of Hamelin', with its potent lesson of keeping one's word, is a story that stayed with Anele from childhood. The piper's brief from the mayor of the town was to get rid of the rats, for which he would be rewarded; when the mayor went back on his word, the piper took the town's children.

'Stories are important because they last,' Anele says. A student leader during the #MustFall movements, Anele is also a law graduate and one of a younger generation of influential South Africans. While not negating the discourses of the past or the value of understanding the many historical factors that shaped their parents' and grandparents' lives, this generation feels strongly that a new narrative is needed. Part of what needs to change, she says, is the language people continue to use to describe black people's experience – words like 'voiceless' and 'defenceless'. 'We need to change that,' she told me.

Seth, who has a passion for reconciliation and, among other things, uses story and song as a facilitator in this field, was moved to tears when he saw the film *Gandhi*, based on Gandhi's life, as a young man. 'It kind of placed me in this space; I was thinking about my youth and who I am. I was serving at that time on a team that was doing youth work. We were doing stuff around justice issues and reconciliation, I think the movie shocked me in a way that I'm also of African and Indian ancestry, and I saw this leader, I saw his life, and maybe what brought me to tears was the journey of truth that he was pursuing, this fight for justice, learning from his time in South Africa. It was connecting me to some of the things I'd lived through. I felt like it was something into my heritage. Later on, I studied more and learned more about the history of indentured labourers in South Africa, between 1890 and 1910, which is my own heritage. Both sides of my family, maternal lines and paternal lines, landed here. Sugarcane plantations were part of it. I think by my reading and writing and learning, I was kind of working out myself. Who am I? Where am I?'

From the first time Seth saw the Gandhi movie, when he was around 20 years old, to watching it again many years later, he said, allowed him to see connectivities. 'My own golden thread started to come out.'

Khayelihle Dominique Gumede's clan, he is proud to acknowledge, are 'the news bringers to the king', and he continues to be an avid absorber and disseminator of knowledge and story. The chief creative officer of Clive Morris Productions, he is passionate about using storytelling for social change. Raised by a single mother, whose influence was strong, he moved around a lot as a child, going to different schools. This necessitated constantly having to reinvent himself and learn new 'codes'. He matriculated as head boy of Parktown Boys' High and counted among his friends many whose parents were intellectuals, artists, activists, social scientists and thinkers. He saw them as the keepers of much wisdom, and he drew on their individual and collective stories and their tradition of lively debate around a table. After beginning a law degree, he realised that his true passion was theatre, its notions of tradition and evolution. 'Creating an imaginative space,' he said, 'where people are able to self-actualise their story,' is empowering.

Steven Mzee likes to draw on powerful biblical stories to illustrate a modern-day phenomenon – for example, to address xenophobia and rejection of 'the foreigner', he retells the story of the good Samaritan, but from the perspective of 'the other', the victim. In framing the story this way, people are able to identify with the victim and understand how he is experiencing the encounter. He has another story, a true one, to illustrate this, which came out of groups in his congregation sharing their stories. It emerged that a white South African conscript who had served in Angola during the Border War, was in the same group as his Angolan age mate. The Angolan man had also served in that same war, but on the other side. The two men discovered that they were in the same territory, in the same week, on the same day. 'We could have killed each other ...' Today they are the best of friends and meet regularly over coffee to chat.

In South Africa, as elsewhere, we are often quick to make assumptions. Zolani Mahola had just dropped her child off at school in Cape Town one morning and found herself standing next to a young white man at the pedestrian crossing, waiting to cross the road while cars ignored the crossing and whizzed past. She looked at him but the man did not make eye contact and said nothing. Zolani dismissed him as 'one of those' until he spoke, after a car had finally stopped to let them walk: 'It's crazy,' he said shyly, 'how few people stop.'

As we cross paths with one another through life, perhaps the pedestrian crossing instructions might be reframed: Stop. Look Left. Look Right. Listen.

PART 3

BELIEVING – HOLDING THE FAITH

Sometimes the future our imagination paints is misty and incomplete and so never amounts to more than a vague longing. Other times our dreams are crushed by reality, like wanting to be a professional soccer player and having lousy hand-eye co-ordination. But sometimes a story burns so brightly in our imagination that in its pursuit we are enabled to push though seemingly insurmountable obstacles.

Sometimes it's a question of holding the faith. Faith is what all of the world's religions require from their followers, and it is through powerful stories that their messages are conveyed most effectively. The greatest influencers in history have intuitively understood and used its power. Martin Luther King, Gandhi and Mandela all painted powerful pictures of freedom and the transformation of unequal societies. Jesus, not only through his storytelling but through the story of his life, death and resurrection, has transformed many lives, mine included.

At a time of deep despair, as a young doctor fresh out of the army and propelled into what to all intents and purposes was a conflict zone, I went through a severe crisis: a psychological breakdown and a doubting of the existence of God. While I made a decision that felt rational, in later years I would continue to experience the constant dissonance of belief and unbelief. But as I swim through the muddy waters of life, they are sometimes clear enough to give me glimpses of the bedrock. The bedrock of truth that gives me hope and direction.

Story, with its profound influence on what we believe and do, can be the conduit for lessons that will hold good for a lifetime and is the thread that transmits values from one generation to another.

I would like to be able to say that it was a period of deep study that awoke me to this truth, but, in reality, I stumbled upon it. And set out, as I recount here in Part 3, without much of a clue, to use story to promote health. I didn't know how I was going to do it – that's partly where holding the faith comes in – but, armed with an idea and a desire to effect change for the good, I trusted that I had two of the key components.

I make no secret of the fact that I struggle with mental health illness. Anxiety and depression and being unable sometimes to see the way forward have plagued me for much of my life. Trusting that there is help at hand and light in darkness can be easier to say than truly believe. During the years of using fictional stories in the pursuit of societal health, I came to realise that when I had the courage to tell my own story, especially my struggles with mental illness, this had the potential to bring healing and hope to others who might be suffering in similar ways. The experience persuaded me to encourage people to share their stories, no matter how ordinary they seem, with others. This sharing of stories has become the heart of one of Heartlines' key projects, 'What's Your Story?', to build empathy and understanding between people.

This theme resonated with many of those I interviewed for this book, which can be clearly seen in 'In Others' Words' at the end of this section.

8.

BUSKER WITH A VISION

People tell me I have a lot of crazy ideas and they're not wrong. One of the craziest was thinking I could sell out the Market Theatre when I was a fourth-year medical student ...

The suburb of Hillbrow, Johannesburg, is another kind of jungle to my East African fantasy – a concrete one – and is considered by many not to be a safe place for the unwary after dark. The tall buildings ensure that evening comes more quickly here. Not wanting to still be trying to find my destination in the dark, I look anxiously up and down the busy street for the Twilight Children sign. In this time of apartheid, Hillbrow is one of the few places where people mix, regardless of race or nationality. It is also a high-water mark at which some of the most marginalised in society, the homeless, the addicted and street children, wash up.

Finally, I find the right door. Tucked between a shop and the entrance to a block of flats, it is protected by a heavy steel gate. I push the adjacent buzzer. This looks more like a prison than a children's home.

After some time, an elderly female voice asks, 'Can I help you?'

'Is that Vivienne?' I ask.

Having established that it is indeed Vivienne, I remind her that I'm the fourth-year medical student who'd called her the previous week. 'You said I should come round?'

Moments later the door swings open and a tired-looking woman with a kind face and hair tied up in a no-nonsense bun, smiles through the gate as she struggles with the lock. Children of various sizes and ages swirl around her. A little girl clings desperately to her leg as two scruffy adolescent boys race past. The noise is deafening. 'Sorry,' she says. 'This is always crazy hour. Dinner time for the little ones and curfew for the children coming off the streets.'

Vivienne shows me around. In a small room, its walls brightly painted with scenes from familiar fairy tales, rows of steel cots are packed together in neat rows. Most are home to at least two and sometimes three babies, ranging in age from a few months to two years. The older children look at me with dull eyes. With extraordinary dexterity a carer is feeding three kids at the same time, balancing a baby and a bottle with one arm and scooping porridge into alternate mouths.

'Most of these children have been abandoned,' Vivienne tells me. 'Their mothers leave them outside our door or people find them and bring them to us. We try to have them adopted or fostered, but the older they get the less hope there is, and they end up living here.' There is sadness in her voice and resignation in her eyes.

'So are those the older kids I've seen?' I ask.

'A few, but a lot of them have been living on the street. It's tragic to hear their stories. Often they've run away to escape abusive parents or they've been kicked out of home when mum or dad finds a new partner.'

I stare silently at this scene. I can't process this. I'm still trying to come to grips with the weight of suffering that medicine has exposed me to. I wonder whether I ever will?

Vivienne leads me to a quieter spot where we sit down in two battered chairs. 'I'm so glad you called,' she says. 'I've been praying for a doctor. We try our best but ...'

'I'm only in fourth year,' I say quickly, but she doesn't seem to hear.

'Perhaps you could come a few times a week? We'll put aside a room for you, but we don't have much money for equipment or medicine. I don't suppose you could provide those ...?'

To be honest, I've not been enjoying the missing chapters in my story, the ones I am living now, that fill in the gap from the idealist boy to hero doctor. I'm having to work damn hard. Eat, sleep, study, repeat. This was unexpected. I'm desperate for the part where I make a real difference and it's very slow in coming. Perhaps I can make a start before I finish medical school and maybe working at Twilight could be that start. But in reality, I know enough to be dangerous and not enough to be useful. As for the money for medicine and equipment, where on earth am I going to find that?

MY FIRST 'CLINIC' throws into stark relief how clueless I am. I make a hash of things even before I start.

'This little boy is wheezing, doctor.'

'I'm not a doctor, just a student,' I correct the carer.

'Yes, doctor,' she responds.

I've never examined let alone undressed a baby and that is where I suffer my first defeat. Baffled by the multitude of clips and frightened by the size and viciousness of the nappy pin, I hesitate long enough for the carer to take over and deftly finish the job. Then all I do is state the obvious and confirm the symptoms. 'Yes, this baby is wheezing.' Then I stammer through some advice, care of the *Reader's Digest*, about cough syrup. The carer is embarrassingly grateful.

And so my clinic continues, a stream of problems from rashes and discharging ears to coughs and colds and all I can do is confirm what they already know. It's a horrible feeling, being out of my depth but having to pretend that I'm not. It's made worse by these people's complete trust in me. I want to run a mile but know I can't. Somehow I am going to need to find a way of doing this properly.

'Properly' involves enlisting the help of some sixth-year medical students – that's the easier part – and raising money, which is going to be much more of a challenge.

I LOVE THE theatre, and especially the Market Theatre, which, in the 1980s, is a quirky, rebellious space in downtown Johannesburg, frequented by wannabee artists, activists and me. My plan is straightforward: book out a performance; sell the tickets; provide some cheese and wine; make a profit. In that order.

Simple.

And in so doing I will have the funds I need to improve things at the Twilight clinic.

I might have been a little short on the planning part. I discover that plays at the Market Theatre are called 'fringe' for a reason. Protest theatre does not sell. Despite fliers, posters and impassioned pleas, there is a week to go and I've sold only a fraction of the tickets I have committed to.

In a break between med school classes I walk over to our usual table in the canteen, where Denis, Megan and Cheryl are already seated.

'How're the ticket sales going, Japh?' Cheryl asks.

I sit down heavily. 'Well, you guys have bought,' I say. 'And so have my mum and dad and a couple of others ...'

'Not well then,' says Megan.

'I think I've sold about 20. Just another 280 to go. I'm stuffed.'

'And the cheese and wine?' Denis asks.

'I was going to use some ticket sales money for that,' I say. 'So at this stage it's going to be more like bread and water. I have so messed this up. Not only am I not raising any money, I'm going to be in a mountain of debt. Guys, I need your help.'

The three of them exchange wry glances. No one seems that surprised. 'Okay, Japh,' Cheryl says with a smile. 'What did you say the name of the play was?'

'*Pula*,' I say. 'I think it's Setswana for rain.' Relief begins to flood over me.

'Sounds beautiful,' says Cheryl. 'Okay – we'd better get selling!'

And sell they do. Parents, near and distant relations, friends of friends. Few, if any, have been to the Market Theatre before. With just a day to go I am elated. We have a full house! This is working out better than I had dared hope.

UP ON STAGE, I look out over the packed theatre, dazzled by the lights but still able to see Denis's parents smiling up at me from the front row. I thank the audience for coming and talk passionately about the Twilight Children and the clinic. 'Enjoy the show!' I conclude to applause and cat-calls from my friends.

This is amazing. I bask in the glow of achievement. Then the performance begins.

'You k...ir b*tch! I'll moer you!' roars the white policeman as he drags a young black woman across the stage. 'I asked you for you bloody pass-book and now you are trying to be clever with me!' He gives her a vicious kick. She screams and wriggles free of his grasp.

There is a collective intake of breath. This is a nice, white, middle-class audience. They are in shock. But this is just the beginning. The next hour is an assault on their senses and their sensibilities, as the horrors of apartheid are dished up with dramatic vigour. The government has been ruthlessly efficient in shielding white people from these realities and tonight's 'entertainment' is an unanticipated ordeal. I can't wait to get out of there and nor can they. But worse is to come.

In a particularly hard-hitting scene filled with expletives and violence, the actor spits at the policeman, except she misses. Almost in slow motion, I see a huge globule of spit arc through the lights and hit Denis's mother square in the face. With careful dignity, she retrieves a hanky from her bag and wipes her face. I wanted to disappear – permanently.

My friends and I reconvene in the canteen the following day.

'Flip, guys, I'm sorry,' I say for the umpteenth time. 'After all you did – and then I screw things up. I should have checked out the play first.'

'And the ticket selling,' Mike laughs.

'Ag, it's fine, Japh,' Cheryl says. 'People knew it was for a good cause.'

'There is a slight complication,' I say slowly. 'I … um … well, apparently I didn't read the contract with the theatre properly. They thought I wanted to book two nights, not one. A week apart. When I told them I didn't want the second night, they weren't sympathetic. They told me it was too late for them to sell the tickets. So, guys, I have a problem. I'm afraid I'm going to need your help again.'

I am aware that it says a lot about me that no one is surprised, but I can see the battle going on within them. We have been friends through thick and thin and we always have each other's backs. This, however, might be a bridge too far.

Denis speaks as if he is in pain. 'Yew, Garth. Um … I don't know. You see … I think we've maxed out our favours.'

'Hang on,' says Megan. 'Wasn't last night the finale? Garth, you—!'

My deception has run out of road.

I give a sheepish grin.

'Garth!' they say in exasperated unison.

ANOTHER NOT-WELL-THOUGHT-through idea is the one I pitch to Aggrey Klaaste a few years later when my day job is at the paediatric unit at Alexandra Clinic.

A doyen of the newspaper world, editor of *The Sowetan* and an influential voice for nation building in the early years of democratic South Africa, Dr Klaaste is a very busy man. I am surprised when he agrees to see me.

I am nervous as I park my car – it feels worse than arriving to write an exam – and being shown into his office doesn't do anything to alleviate my anxiety. On the walls, between several framed front pages that have marked our country's history are honorary doctorates, awards – lots of them – and a large picture of Dr Klaaste hand in hand with Nelson Mandela. Now I'm properly intimidated.

Aggrey Klaaste rises from behind his desk. I see a compact man, late middle age, receding dark hair speckled with grey. His heavy thick-lensed glasses remind me of my dad. I'm sure that when he removes them there will be a dent in the bridge of his nose. He smiles broadly and shakes my hand. 'Dr Japhet? Come and take a seat. How can I help you?'

'Dr Klaaste,' I say, with a lot more confidence than I suddenly feel,

'I'd like to write for your newspaper.' He smiles. I guess he's heard this before. I continue quickly. 'My idea is to have a weekly column to make health information accessible to the everyman …' I trail off, but he nods, encouraging me to continue. 'Er … you see, Dr Klaaste … as a doctor working in Alex, I've become so aware that much of what I see is preventable … and it breaks my heart.'

'Yes—'

'Okay, well …' I hesitate, then say, 'Let me give you an example. Just yesterday I was on casualty duty when I was called over to see a patient. He was a man in late middle age. I didn't need to examine him to know that he had a bleed into his brain. His right arm was hanging lifelessly off the side of the bed. The desperate look in his eyes and the fact that he couldn't speak confirmed my diagnosis for me. His distraught wife told me that years earlier he had been diagnosed with high blood pressure but despite her pleas, he had refused to take medication. This was the result. So tragic. So preventable.'

Dr Klaaste is clearly moved by my story. 'I lost my dad to a stroke and I have high blood pressure,' he murmurs quietly. 'So what are you suggesting?'

'I would try and help a man like that understand what high blood pressure is and why it needs long-term treatment. My idea would be to have a question and answer column in the paper where I would use stories to explain things.'

'I get it,' he says. 'So what sort of story would you tell?'

'So in this case, I might have a fictional Mrs Sithole from Diepkloof in Soweto write to me like this: "Dear Doctor, the clinic says my husband has very high blood pressure. They say unless he takes pills every day, he will die. He says he won't take the pills because he feels just fine. He's such a stubborn man, doctor, what should I do?"'

Dr Klaaste chuckles. 'I'm a stubborn man myself,' he admits. 'Go on. I'm curious to know how you would respond.'

True to form, I have not prepared for this part. I think quickly.

'Um … ah … I think I would respond something like this: "Dear Mrs Sithole. Thank you for your question. I would like to explain high blood pressure to you by telling you a story. Imagine there is a very full minibus taxi. The driver stops at the garage for petrol but also asks the attendant to pump up the tyres. The attendant is having a really bad day and puts far too much air into the tyres. The driver pulls back onto the road. His taxi feels fine, just like it was before he stopped, but suddenly – Bwah! A tyre bursts, the taxi skids and then rolls and rolls. Many passengers are injured and some are killed. You see, Mrs Sithole, the blood in our veins is like the air in a car tyre. If the pressure of the blood gets too high, the veins in our head can burst and we get a 'stroke', which we can die from. The scary thing is that just like the taxi driver couldn't tell that the pressure in his tyres was too high, we often feel fine until suddenly – Bwah! we have a stroke. That's why you need to get your husband to take his pills." I'd end off by thanking her for her question.'

I stop. Just listening to myself makes me question my idea. Dr Klaaste says nothing. He makes a steeple of his fingers; he looks deep in thought. He is a kind man so he's probably working out how to let me down gently. But instead he smiles at me and says warmly, 'I like it. Your storytelling could do with a polish, and I warn you, you may have threats from the taxi industry, but I think the concept could work. How about a weekly column? Perhaps we could call it "The Healthy Nation"?'

I'm in shock. He likes it! 'That would be great,' I say.

As he sees me out, he says, 'Get your typed column to us by Thursday each week. And we'll see how it goes.'

Another thing I hadn't foreseen. 'I can't type,' I confess, even as I know this isn't his problem.

'Just hand write it then,' says Dr Klaaste. 'Linda will type it up.'

Linda is Dr Klaaste's PA, who has been nothing but friendly and welcoming so far. I fear she might be less so when she sees my handwriting – think the love child of hieroglyphics and Hebrew – and I feel a wave of advance sympathy for her. I've always suspected that the main reason I scraped through med school was that my lecturers, unable to decipher my scrawl, gave me the benefit of the doubt.

Fortunately for me, Linda proves resilient and somehow I manage to produce the weekly advice column. I have plenty of material to draw on from the clinic and the story form has always appealed to me and felt effective. The transformative power of words and stories, even though I may not have realised it, has been at work in my life for many years.

I'M SITTING ALONE on a pavement in Melville. It is still warm from the heat of the day; I shift my backside, trying, futilely, for a softer piece of concrete. I'm careful not to spill my beer. Not sure if it's my second or third, but it's the Mardi Gras, so I'm not counting.

It's that lovely time of day where the light goes amber, rendering everything golden. The scent of cooking wors and dope drifts on the air. Dope's not my thing, but I could do with a wors roll. As I stand in line to buy one, music of different cultures clashes and mingles – folk, Afrobeat, acoustic, hip hop and stuff I don't recognise, all providing an appropriate backdrop to this suburban street party.

Clusters of noisy, happy partyers ebb and flow down the street. Rainbow? Fruit salad? What best summarises the variations in age, culture, gender, race? I don't know. Anyway, most of them look like they have it together. They're enjoying the now and don't seemed too bothered about the future. How I wish I could be like them. But I can't. The beer's taking the edge off my angst but still the 'What's next, Garth?' question keeps ricocheting around my skull.

I'm okay for now. Doctor running the paeds clinic in Alex. I've no vision for what's next, though, and it's freaking me out.

Specialise in paediatrics? I love working with kids, but if I'm honest, the thought 'I'm so desperate for sleep that I couldn't care if the child dies' is not compatible with paediatrics.

Ophthalmology? Love the idea. Good hours, massive need in Africa, and I could make a real difference. But my hands shake and I'm easily distracted, so, um, no.

So what then?

I'm feeling distinctly mellow as I sip my third or is it fourth beer? Red sauce oozes from the roll onto my hand and drips down onto the pavement. Suddenly my scattered thoughts crystallise and my heart jumps. The phone call I received yesterday has sparked an idea.

'Garth, it's Linda. Just thought I would let you know that your column is doing so well. Our readers seem to really love it. In fact, on the day it's published, our circulation jumps by 10 per cent.'

'Wow, that amazing!' I said. 'But don't you think that's because you also publish the horseracing section that day?'

I can hear the smile in her voice. 'We don't think that's it. In fact, we think your column's a hit and we would really like you to continue.'

Yes. To continue. That's it, that's the idea. But what if …?

I take another slug of beer.

What if instead of just using the newspaper, which only reaches a few people, we could tell the same stories through a different medium? On radio. Maybe even TV? At prime time. People love medical dramas. Perhaps I could start a medical drama with a purpose? Maybe the same themes could run across radio, TV *and* print? I could reach millions of people!

Now my mind is really racing.

It could run for years, and deal with different issues over time. This is such a fabulous idea! Visions of people glued to their radios, gathered around their TV sets and poring over beautifully illustrated publications compete with images of me running an organisation and loving it.

'I'm so sorry, didn't see you there.'

The inebriated shatterer of my dreams staggers away, having knocked the warm beer, which splatters all over me, and the remnants of my wors roll from my hands.

I didn't see you there. What he would have seen if he'd looked was a slightly sozzled 27-year-old doctor having an existential crisis.

But I can't shake the idea. Long after my hangover has worn off, my dream, and with it my excitement, grows. I hang onto it with the tenacity of a drowning man. It feels like I finally have a vision for my future. I share it with whomever will listen. Most people are kind. They listen to me and make encouraging noises – 'Great idea', 'Good luck' – but no one is offering to help. Some people think the idea is an especially crazy one, even for me.

'You want to do what?'

'Make a hit TV and radio drama.'

'Ja, sure. And where would you begin? Where would the money come from?'

I know that this time I'm going to have to do better than sell out a couple of performances at the Market Theatre. I can't let this go. I won't let this go. But I have no idea what to do next. There is no map, no instruction manual.

Gradually I become worn down and my initial excitement is replaced by the familiar rising black tide. The doubting me replaces the dreaming me. Like a drug addict coming down from a high, I crash back into despair.

I am rescued by Jim from Beth Shalom's words of advice for when the path ahead is not clear. What was it he'd said?

'Just wait for the next cat's eye in the road.'

I AM BACK in Aggrey Klaaste's office at *The Sowetan*, but this time he is not alone. He introduces me as 'our newest journalist, Garth Japhet' and invites me to take a seat. While Aggrey might be the visionary nation builder, MD Rory Wilson is all business. He is the man responsible for making a profit and paying the bills. He may have a kindly demeanour but I note the unmistakable 'I'm no bleeding heart' look in his eye.

Aggrey gets right to it. 'I believe you have a new idea,' he says to me. 'I'm intrigued.'

I proceed to describe my vision. Phew, it's really a long shot. They listen intently. When I'm finished, Aggrey smiles at me. 'Garth,' he says, passion in his voice, 'if we are going to realise the potential of our beautiful land and give us hope for our better future, we are going to have to do things differently.'

My heart sinks a little.

'That's why I love your idea,' says Aggrey. To my astonishment the MD is nodding in agreement.

'How can we help you?' Rory asks.

As I step out into daylight and walk to my car I wonder if I look as dazed and amazed as I feel. Did what just happened really happen? Did *The Sowetan* just agree to pay my salary for three months *and* host a lunch with the head of the TV station CCTV (later to become SABC 1) at South Africa's public broadcaster so that I can pitch my idea to them? I can scarcely believe it.

A CAT'S EYE in the road is one thing. The potholes beyond are quite another. It is probably just as well I can't see those.

I've lost count of the number of advertising executives I've met with in the last few months. They all look much the same – designer jeans, form-hugging shirt, snake-skin shoes (although I'm not sure about the snake-skin) – and they all say much the same things.

'Dr Japhet, so nice to meet you, I absolutely love your idea, let me chat to some colleagues and I'll get right back to you …'

I've got used to the chrome and leather furniture, the hip people who come and go, all looking stressed and important, as I wait to be summoned. I've got used to the not-a-hair-out-of-place receptionists, the high-end biscuits and proper coffee. I could also get used to rejection but these guys don't even come back to me. Time and money to get my vision for a medical drama series going are running out and my spirits are beginning to run low.

I've knocked on so many doors, talked to so many people and I've drawn a big, fat blank. I've got no clue who else to approach. I wake up at 3am, my mind at war with itself. If not this, then what? My fear of being directionless is compounded by my terror of descending back into depression.

My state of mind is not helped by the nagging anxiety about the future of our country. Without some miracle it seems like we are headed for a civil war. The daily flow of brutalised bodies I've seen in casualty at the clinic in Alex seems to make this possibility even more real. All this energy and angst for a country that I might have to flee from? God help me. As the day lightens, my need to get moving wrenches me out of my circular thoughts.

At the clinic I fall into the familiar routine of the paediatric unit. I am busy with a patient one morning when Sister Theresa puts her head through the cubicle curtains. 'Sorry to disturb, ma,' she says to the patient. 'Garth – there is a package for you.' She hands me an A4 envelope with 'Dr Garth Japhet – By Hand' written on it in bold type. I'm not expecting any package, certainly not a hand-delivered one. What could it be – a summons, an insurance policy? I put the envelope down and return to my patient. 'Don't worry, ma,' I tell the anxious mother, 'your son's cough will improve quickly. Just make sure that he takes the medicine three times a day until the packet is finished.'

When I find a moment to take a breath I tear open the mysterious envelope. It contains a neat ring-bound document with a label on the front:

> Proposal to Dr Garth Japhet
> for the production of a 13-part hospital drama
> From Hannelie Pieterse, Philo Pieterse Productions

The note attached requests a meeting.

I don't even know what a production company is. That's how little I know.

In her high heels and wearing one of those 'power suits' I've only ever seen in magazines, Hannelie Pieterse is the essence of chic. She has auburn hair and is beautifully made up. And she is charming.

'Thank you so much for coming, Dr Japhet,' she says.

I nod, bemused (like I might have turned down the invitation!).

'A friend of mine in the advertising industry told me about your idea for a TV series. I hope you don't mind that we took the liberty of putting together a proposal for you?'

'I don't mind,' I say, trying my best to look cool.

'We think that we are the ideal production partners for you,' she goes on. 'We have years of experience in drama and, more recently, educational television.'

Hannelie Pieterse is pitching to *me*. It's not easy to look cool when excitement is threatening to break through the dark clouds like a ray of sunlight, but I do what I hope is a passable impression. As she continues, adding shape and ideas to what until now has only been a vision in my head, describing how they might turn it into a reality that will entertain as well as educate millions of viewers, I can hardly believe it. It all sounds too good to be true.

But it is good. And it is true. Philo Pieterse Productions will prove to be ideal partners.

Soul City is going to happen.

But it's by no means plain sailing.

I WRAP MY hands around my mug of tea, trying to warm them. It's cold this morning and there is no heating in the clinic's tea room. I take a seat next to my colleague Grant Rex. We've known each other since our student days when Grant was a bearded student activist. He's now a bearded doctor.

'How's the project going, Garth?' he asks. I know he is genuinely interested, so I bring him up to speed.

'It's going, Grant,' I tell him. 'As to where, though, I'm still not sure.'

Grant smiles. Like me, he's something of an idealist.

'When I'm feeling positive, I really think this thing could work. I've had these amazing breakthroughs, like this production company that just appeared – I told you about Philo Pieterse Productions, right? And South Africa's leading scriptwriter, Richard Beynon, has agreed to write the series. Unreal! Then I stumble upon this innovative publishing company, Jacana, and they are going to do the publications.'

I pause to grab a sandwich, which promptly disintegrates. While I am scooping up crumbs Grant asks, 'What does Tim think?'

Tim Wilson is our director, a tall slender paediatrician with grey hair and flowing beard. He could have played Gandalf in *Lord of the Rings*. Not only has Tim transformed Alex Clinic into a model for good primary health care, but he is also seriously connected.

'Tim's been amazing. He's even managed to get me another grant to stretch my three months to six.'

'That's cool, Garth,' Grant says. 'Sounds like things are really cooking.'

'Ja,' I sigh, 'but I've no idea how I'm going to find the R5 million I need. Right now I'm down to R20 000, and it's disappearing fast.' Just saying this out loud makes me have a wobble.

Grant gives me a sympathetic smile. 'Sorry, can't help you there, dude … Wish you luck.'

And then I tell him how I'm really feeling. I tell him that I'm not sure I can do this. After a year by myself on the Soul City project, I confide, I'm about ready to call it quits. A serious look comes over Grant's face. 'Ah, now *there* I think I may be able to help you,' he says.

The 'help' comes in the form of Dr Shereen Usdin.

She walks purposefully into my cubicle and sits down, bangles clinking. I do not recognise her. She is slightly older than me. She wears her hair in a brown bob and has passionate eyes.

'You must be Garth,' she says.

I nod, taken aback. I had been expecting a coughing/vomiting/malnourished child to be next in my cubicle … not this woman, who is smiling broadly at me as if she has something important to impart. 'I'm Shereen,' she says, as if that should explain it. 'Grant's friend.'

We exchange pleasantries. I'm still not sure why she is here.

'Grant has told me what you're trying to do and I think it's the most fantastic idea,' she says. 'Look, I know this is weird, but I'm coming to join you. Even if you can't pay me.'

I'm stunned. I really don't know what to say, so I don't say anything.

Shereen hurries on. 'I know this is crazy,' she says, 'but this is *exactly* what I've been looking for.'

If I had foresight, Shereen would be exactly who I would look for. We complement each other. She is seriously smart and fluent in public health-speak like 'social mobilisation' and 'self-efficacy', whereas I'm just a beginner. She can use a computer. I can't. She is politically astute. I'm not.

So now we are two. I'm a lone nut no more, and it feels very good to share the space.

It also feels like a real God-incidence.

9.

THE GREATEST STORY

The man sitting opposite me does not look like a priest. No white collar or dangling cross. Dressed in an art-meets-fashion type of way, in fact, Brian looks more like a middle-aged advertising executive. I later learn that's exactly what he used to be.

'Coffee?' Brian asks.

'Please,' I stammer. This feels like a big mistake.

'Sugar?'

'No, thanks, just milk.'

Brian sits down in a chair worn comfortable by many years of use and proceeds to prepare coffee in two chipped mugs. As he mixes and stirs, my foggy mind reflects on the last week.

It started with a visit to a psychiatrist, a kindly man who confirmed my diagnosis – which I have for years simply labelled Stuffed Head Syndrome (SHS). I have anxiety, depression and have suffered a breakdown. The psychiatrist prescribed a fearsome cocktail of antidepressants, anxiolytics and sleeping tablets. 'You might feel worse before you feel better, but in the meantime, hang in there,' he said.

He was right. I feel weird, sort of fuzzy and disconnected. So much so that on one of my ward rounds a nurse pointed out that I was examining the same patient for the second time. A nice new symptom to add to my current ones of hopelessness and despair, both markers of my existential crisis.

As I see it, I have only two options. I must either end it all or come up with a plan to make sense of my life and try to chart a way forward.

I have been wrapped in a cloak of blackness and despair. My thoughts endlessly reprocess and always with the same result: there is no way out. For me this is a special horror. No matter how bad things have been there was always the next step, but not this time. To make matters worse, I have no reasons for my despair. I have had a privileged upbringing; my parents are still together; I have never been abused or bullied; and I have had a great education. Pull yourself together is what I tell myself. But I can't. Pounding heart, fast thoughts but slow words, and tiredness – oh, such tiredness, so tired that it's an effort to move.

But to the outside world – the curse of the mentally ill – I look perfectly healthy.

To my mind there are two options. The first I am not ready to take (beside which, I lack the courage), so I take the second. This is to consult professionals. My plan is threefold. First I will see a psychiatrist, then a careers counsellor and then a priest. The psychiatrist, as I have said, confirmed my diagnosis and prescribed medication. The careers counsellor listens attentively as I say, 'I've given up medicine and enrolled in an MBA,' then persuades me that nine years of study and practice can still be salvaged. I can still find a path in medicine, she suggests.

The priest, Brian, is my third call. He hands me my coffee.

My hand trembles when I take the mug and coffee slops on the table as I set it down. 'I'm sorry,' I say, hoping he hasn't seen the tremor, but he just smiles and says, 'No problem.' And then, 'How can I help you?'

After giving him a few quick facts – age, profession and so on – I launch into a series of disjointed questions and half-answers. 'Is there any meaning to this life? Because I'm not sure there is …' 'Does God exist? Because if He does, He either doesn't care and can't be trusted or He's got a sick sense of humour …' And a bunch of other existential questions that are currently bouncing around my stuffed head. I'm desperate and angry.

The priest leans forward, listening intently, not interrupting my frustrated flow of words. When I finally stop for breath, he says, 'Perhaps before I start to answer some of your questions, you could tell me what has precipitated this crisis?'

I pause. Try to get my thumping heart and rapid breathing under control.

'Take your time,' he says. 'I am in no hurry. Tell me what's going on.'

And so I do.

THE YEAR IS 1990. Nelson Mandela has only just been released and so have I, from the army. I have gone back to the place I love most, KwaZulu-Natal, to pursue my dream of rural medicine.

I'm on the fourth floor of Edendale Hospital, a sprawling face-brick complex set on a lush, hut-strewn hill in the Edendale valley just outside Pietermaritzburg. Edendale is the major referral hospital for the whole of the KwaZulu-Natal Midlands. That is, if you're black.

'Guys, quickly! You have got to see this! Now!'

Dave, a medical officer in obstetrics, is standing by the window of the doctors' tea room, gesturing wildly. It's clear from the urgency in his voice that now means now and so, trailing flapping white coats and holding half-eaten sandwiches, we converge on the window. Dave is pointing across the valley at the opposite hill. 'This can't be happening!'

A ragged line of ant-like figures are running down the grassy slope, trailing puffs of smoke. We open the window and hear the distant pop-pop-pop of their guns and see the flash of sunlight on steel. They're herding people before them and between the gunfire we hear distant screams. 'It's no longer just happening up the valley,' I say. 'God help them ...'

For the last few days the news has been full of what the media will later dub 'the seven-day war'. A simmering conflict between Inkatha-aligned warlords and ANC comrades has burst into flame. Inkatha's impis have been systematically 'cleansing' the valley, driving the old, the infirm, women and children before them. Anyone left behind is maimed or slaughtered. An island of refuge is St Raphael Catholic Church, a sleepy mission station in the middle of the valley. When it opened its gates overnight it was flooded with over 15 000 scared, injured and hungry people. The frightening thing is that I'm the doctor responsible for them.

The phone rings. 'Garth, there is a gentleman asking for the doctor in charge of community health – it's for you,' Dave says. I take the receiver from him.

'Hello, Dr Japhet speaking.'

'Doctor,' says a deep male voice, 'it's Father Dlamini speaking. I'm the priest at St Raphael's. Please, I believe you can help us …' The next words come out in a rush. 'We're drowning, I've got many, many people, some are badly hurt and others are sick, I don't know what to do—'

Ice filters into my chest. I'm already not in a great space and now this.

There is no back-up. It is just me. Hospitals expect people to come to them not vice versa. I'm not sure what to do, but I decide to try to make it through to the mission station and see what's going on there.

I get into my old silver Jetta and head up the valley. The road is really quiet, no people, just a few unconcerned goats grazing here and there; they seem to be the only living things without fear right now.

A few kilometres up, the road is blocked by a collection of intimidating mud-brown vehicles. I recognise them as Casspirs (my recent two – and only – weeks of army training weren't a complete waste!). Three cold-faced soldiers signal for me to stop and get out of the car.

'Where are you going?' one of them asks in heavily accented English.

'I'm a doctor from Edendale,' I tell the man. 'I am trying to get to St Raphael's. The priest has called for help … I believe there are many injured people up there.'

The men turn to each other and proceed to have a rapid interchange in Portuguese. So this is the infamous 32 Battalion, mercenaries from Angola – not to be messed with.

'You can't go further, it's too dangerous,' the first man says.

I hesitate, swallow. I'm conflicted. Isn't this why I wanted to be a doctor? To be heroic, to save against the odds? My body is screaming *You are not cut out for danger!* while my mind is saying, *If you don't do this now, then what has this whole crazy thing been about? You gritted it out through med school so you could live your dream. This is your dream.* I take a deep breath.

'I have to go,' I tell him.

More rapid Portuguese. Then the soldier who seems to be in charge says, 'Okay, we'll escort you.'

I get back in the car and continue my journey up the valley, this time sandwiched in by two Casspirs. More silent kilometres pass, punctuated only by smouldering huts and wandering cows. It's eerie. There is not a soul to be seen. Suddenly, as we come round a bend there is St Raphael's, a swarm of figures clustered around the church's mustard-coloured walls.

'We'll wait for you here,' the lieutenant says as we arrive at the gates.

I thank him, park and walk towards the church buildings. It feels like every square inch of the grounds is covered. Bundles of clothes, cooking pots and bedding compete for space with people of every age, size and shape. The only thing they all have in common are the expressions that are all too evident on their faces – desperation, shock and despair.

In this crowd I definitely stand out. White guy, white coat. All eyes are on me. I approach an elderly man who is sitting on the building's step. He looks up at me with cataract-filled eyes.

'Sawubona, mkhulu,' I greet him.

'Sawubona, dokotela,' he replies.

'Mkhulu, ukuphi umfundisi?' I enquire.

He says the priest is in the church. I thank him and head in that direction.

There does not seem to be much difference between inside and outside in terms of the numbers of people, except that while outside is bright, inside there is only the dappled light from the stained-glass windows. It streams over the mass of people that fill every available space. Just below the altar, I see the priest in his cream cassock seated at a table. There is an elderly nun with him. From the line of people queuing up in front of them, it looks like they are trying to document the refugees. As I walk towards the table, two children crash into my legs; they laugh and scamper away. For a moment I'm astonished. In the midst of all of this, children are playing?

The priest rises to greet me. I see a man who is probably in his mid-40s. He is powerfully built but he looks wilted, and his eyes tell of a period of great strain and sleeplessness.

'You must be Dr Garth?' he says. 'Thank you for coming.'

'How can I help you, Father?' I ask.

'I am not sure,' he responds. 'There are only four of us, me and three sisters, and we're just battling to establish some order here, let alone feed the people and care for those who need care.'

My heart goes out to him. In the same way that medical school had not prepared me for this, I doubt that seminary had prepared him. From quiet rural church to refugee camp in 24 hours. I'm not sure anything could have prepared either of us.

'Where have you placed the sick?' I ask.

In answer he says only, 'Come with me' and beckons me to follow him. We walk into a small adjoining room. My eyes adjust to the gloom. What I see makes the previous scenes look positively ordered. The floor is covered with a tangle of bodies. There are cries, whispers and groans emanating from the group of mainly young men. Even in this light, I can see a variety of horrific wounds. The savagery inflicted by pangas exposing internal organs and bleeding muscle contrasts with the neat holes of bullet wounds.

It's overwhelming and I am overwhelmed. I have no supplies with me and a doctor without equipment is like a car without a motor, pretty useless.

'I'll see whether I can get army ambulances to take the worst of these patients to Edendale,' I tell Father Dlamini, 'and then I will come back tomorrow. I'll also let the crisis committee know how desperate things are here. I know they are working on a plan to send food and help.'

With the relief of a burden shared, Father Dlamini gives me a small smile. 'Thank you,' he says. 'It feels better just to know that people know.'

As I make to leave, my eyes are drawn to the corner of the room where a small elderly lady is stooped over a figure on the floor. His smiling face and overly large head contrast with his slight, deformed body. His thin legs are permanently crossed. Permanently because I can see the rope-like contractures that will prevent any attempt to move them. This is wounding of a different kind, not from the barrel of a gun or the tip of a spear, but from deprivation of oxygen at birth.

Father Dlamini follows my gaze. 'They arrived this morning,' he says. 'Theirs is an extraordinary story. His name is Bongani, he's 23. His mother abandoned him at birth and left him with his grandmother. Last night, when their homestead was attacked, she hid him the long grass. She stayed with him till morning and then, too afraid to go home, she walked the 10 kilometres down the valley to the mission with Bongani on her back.'

I find this hard to believe. Even in his shrunken state, Bongani is much bigger than his grandmother. And yet it is true. The depth of his grandmother's love had given her the strength and the courage to bring him here. Of everything I have seen today this moves me the most.

'I'm going to try to help them,' I say.

It will take me a while, but eventually I will succeed in getting Bongani into a wonderful place of care for the first time in his life. There will be deep satisfaction in this.

'PHEW, THAT IS quite some story,' Brian says. 'I saw news reports about the seven-day war. It must have been very traumatic.'

'It was,' I acknowledge, and we both fall silent.

'I believe Nelson Mandela visited that mission station? Did you meet him?"

'Yes, I did. In fact, it was a few days after that first visit to St Raphael's. I started a clinic there, just to do what I could. He walked in unannounced while I was working, flanked by his bodyguards. I stood up, quite shocked, and the first thing I thought was, wow, you're so much taller than I imagined. He was amazing, wanted to know what the situation was. I was struck by how he really listened to me, a junior doctor, I mean really listened.'

'The mark of a great leader,' Brian says. 'You're fortunate to have met him.'

'I know.'

'But clearly something happened?' Brian prompts. 'As that was a few weeks back and now you're here. In Johannesburg.'

'Yes. I had to come home. I wasn't in a great space, even before that happened. I was feeling like everything that I had worked for and sacrificed was for nothing. I've resigned myself to accepting that this world is a seriously stuffed-up place and that my childish dreams of "making a difference" are just that – childish. Maybe there is no God and no purpose. Maybe we are just evolved animals and it's the survival of the fittest, and anyone who thinks otherwise, including me, is a fool. So that senseless violence, that suffering and heartache … it sent me over the edge. I couldn't sleep, couldn't think straight. All I could see was blackness and pointlessness ahead. So I left. I felt awful leaving the situation, but I could do nothing else.'

Brian looks at me with calm concern. 'And so you are looking for answers,' he says.

'Yes,' I say with a sigh.

In the frustrating manner of the wise, Brian prevaricates. 'I'm not sure about the answers,' he says, 'but I can try to help you think through your questions.' I nod, but I'm disappointed.

'Has God ever been real in your life? I'm asking because I sense you may have had a faith once. Am I right?'

'Real enough to trust that God had supernaturally set me on this path,' I respond bitterly, 'only to find that this seems to be some sort of cosmic joke.'

Brian is unfazed by my anger. 'And what made you think He was real?'

'Because of what I can only describe as a miracle.'

'Tell me about it,' he says.

'When I was eleven, I was sent on a Christian camp, why, I'm not sure.

Mum was a part-time Anglican and maybe she thought I should get a dose of religion. So I went to this camp in the Magaliesberg full of trepidation. I battled to spend one night away from home with friends, let alone four nights with a bunch of strangers.'

'And?' Brian prompts.

'It was awful! I find this so hard to explain, but, for no reason at all, I was homesick from the moment I arrived. All the other kids were playing and laughing and I just sat on the sidelines in tears, begging them to call my parents to come and fetch me. Then this young guy comes up to me and asks me to come and sit with him on a bench away from the rest. He put his arm around my shoulders and started to pray, asking Jesus to become real to me and give me peace. And—' I pause as I vividly remember the moment, 'and, well, I can only describe what happened as a miracle, because from that moment not only did all anxiety leave me but I was filled with joy, like I had been given a mega dose of fast-acting Prozac. That snivelling homesick boy was instantly transformed. The rest of the camp was surreal.'

'And when you got home?' Brian asks.

'It continued,' I tell him. 'I was a real pain. I couldn't stop telling my sceptical parents what God had done.' Brian chuckles.

'But after a time the experience started to fade and my anxieties returned with a vengeance. I was left with just enough faith to believe that God had touched my life. And so when I got into medicine I thought, this is a God thing; it's meant to be. This is what He means me to do with my life. And then I find it's not. And now I wish that God had left me alone and that the "miracle" had never happened. There is a part of me that envies people who are comfortable with a see and touch life, one with no greater meaning or spiritual dimension.'

'And the other part of you?' Brian asks, curious.

'Knows that we are more than a physical body. Every time I've been present when someone dies, I have sensed that something has left their body. I don't know, it's hard to explain … but maybe not so much to someone in your line of work,' I say wryly.

'The spirit.' Brian chuckles.

'Ja, and if that is real, then there must be something more to this life.' Brian looks at me sympathetically.

'I know you don't feel favoured right now,' he says, 'but many people go their whole lives without experiencing the presence of God in such a dramatic way, nor have they had evidence of the spiritual dimension.'

If this is favour, God can keep it, I think to myself, but Brian is waiting for me to go on. 'I staked my life's decisions on believing that God exists,' I say, 'that He is good, despite the pain in the world, and that He has a plan for my life. Only to find that it isn't true.'

After a considered pause, Brian says, 'It's not surprising you feel dreadful. You're dealing with the pain of the loss of your belief in your purpose and feeling betrayed by the author of that belief.'

I nod miserably. That pretty much sums it up.

'Don't you think it's too soon to know whether your trust in God is misplaced?' Brian suggests. 'My feeling is that you're still at the beginning of your story and you are judging the author before you see the final chapter.' I shift in my seat; part of me wants to believe him.

'Well, unless it has an unexpected twist in the tail, I've a pretty good sense of the ending,' I say.

I feel utterly despondent as I say this. Lack of hope for one's future is surely one of man's most painful conditions.

Brian looks at me as if he's waiting for more. Sensing there is no more, he seems intuitively to know that in order to help me, a concrete approach to my current dilemma is what is needed. He speaks slowly.

'I think that your future comes down to exploring whether your decision to believe that God is both good and that you have understood His purpose for your life was rational.'

'I suppose so,' I say. 'Sort of blue pill, red pill. If I decide I've screwed up, then I abandon the current script; if I haven't, then I hang in there and continue to trust that this story will end well?'

He's momentarily confused and then brightens. '*The Matrix*?' he asks.

We laugh, relieved to break the gloom.

'In essence, it comes down to a single question,' says Brian. 'Is there evidence that God is good and trustworthy? Because if He is, then He won't have led you astray.'

I concede that this makes sense. 'But how can we know the answer to that question other than through our own experiences?' I ask. 'Mine don't point in that direction.'

'Because we can review the evidence and make a perfectly rational decision without committing intellectual suicide. Faith, like love, can begin in a feeling, but then it needs to be a decision that can anchor your life regardless of circumstances and emotion.'

Just then a bee alights on the edge of my coffee mug. I've never been stung but my sister almost died from a bee sting once and I'm not taking any chances. I jump up and make a hasty exit, leaving Brian sitting open-mouthed. Just when he felt he was getting through to me! From the safety of the doorway, I apologise. 'Sorry! I think I may be allergic.'

When Brian realises it's the bee I'm referring to and not our conversation, he is relieved. He ushers the bee out the window and I come back in and sit down.

'You had me worried! Shall we continue?'

'Please,' I say, the adrenalin having cleared my head.

'To contemplate the life of Jesus and his teachings is to know the nature of God,' Brian says. 'If we believe, as we do, that Jesus was God in human form it makes sense to observe what Jesus did and pay attention to what he said. Don't you think?'

'I suppose so,' I say tentatively.

'Well, then, I want you to hear the story of Jesus as if you are hearing it for the first time. Try to put aside the image of the sanitised Jesus you're familiar with and listen afresh.'

'Okay,' I say. 'I'll try.'

'The real Jesus was a radical who shocked the establishment. In today's society, he would be labelled a troublemaker and a maverick, for he was not afraid to speak truth to power or to befriend and embrace the most marginalised in society – the poor, lepers, prostitutes and tax collectors. Yes, he was the great peacemaker but he could also show righteous anger, like when he whipped the money-changers out of the Temple.'

'So not gentle Jesus meek and mild?' I say wryly.

'Not at all. CS Lewis describes God so well with his allegory in *The Lion, the Witch and the Wardrobe.* "Course he isn't safe. But he's good." But it wasn't just what Jesus did that shook things up, it was what he said. He preached the most bizarre message. Turn the other cheek when wronged. Love, don't hate, your enemies. The meek and the poor, not the rich and powerful, will be first in God's kingdom. It's what some have called the "upside-down kingdom" because it turns our concept of what's important in life on its head. That the world honours and cares for the marginalised and disenfranchised is a direct result of the event two thousand years ago when God took the side of the victim. A fact that would surprise many in the social justice movement.'

'And right-wing Christians,' I say grimly. 'I can never understand how they are moved to righteous anger by the fate of the unborn child but seem less interested in the plight of the vulnerable born. It baffles and angers me.'

'Agreed,' Brian says, then continues. 'If you were ambitious or mad enough to want to launch a religion and needed to concoct a story to get people to subscribe to it, Jesus' story is not going to be the one you'd choose. The life and message of Jesus was so counter-cultural, so different to the all-conquering messiah expected by the Jews, that the fact that it spread from an unknown corner of a minor territory to influence human history like no other defies belief. That is, unless it's true.'

'I get it. That Jesus' story seems so bizarre that it points to truth,' I say. 'But that doesn't necessarily mean that Jesus was God.'

'True – but there is a part two to his story, an unexpected ending, which is the event on which the answer to your questions hinges.'

'The resurrection.'

'Exactly. If the resurrection happened, then Jesus is who he said he was, and everything he said and did was true. If it didn't, then those of us who believe are fools.'

'And you think there is evidence that he rose again?'

'I do. We need to look no further than at the lives of the disciples after the resurrection. Here was a group of men, peasants, most of them, who had left everything to follow the man they believed to be the Messiah, the son of God. Then, like an ordinary mortal, Jesus is arrested and killed. So naturally they attempt to dissociate themselves from him lest they suffer the same fate. But then something happens that transforms them from men on the run to fearless preachers willing to be persecuted and killed for their beliefs. Why? What would do that? What possible upside could there be to suffering and dying for something you know to be a lie? And yet that is what they did. They must have experienced the risen Christ. There does not seem to be any other logical explanation.'

Brian sits back and lets the silence rest between us. I have heard the evidence and now I realise that I need to make a decision. Blue pill, red pill.

I'm still struggling, so I say, with youthful righteousness, 'If it's true, why does faith seem to make so little difference to the way people live their lives?' Brian nods in sympathy.

'I think it's because the life that the real Jesus calls us to seems too uncomfortable and too risky. And because many believe that Jesus' main instruction was to redeem people's souls so as to get them into heaven. They believe that people's material situation is less important than getting them right with God.'

'Blows my mind,' I say. 'That's not the essence of the story you've just told me. Surely it's both souls and material conditions?'

'Of course it is. But we have always cherry-picked which part of Jesus' life and teachings we want to follow. The apartheid theologians are a case in point.'

'And pain? Good God, suffering world? That contradiction?' Brian nods.

'The great theologian GK Chesterton calls them "furious opposites", which Christianity has got over the difficulty of by keeping them both and keeping them both furious. Perhaps pain is the greatest mystery that keeps many people from God. I believe God grieves with us. He calls us to be his hands and feet in a fallen world. But perhaps that's a discussion for another time?'

I'm struggling. I know whatever decision I make will determine my future because it needs to be all or nothing. Although I'm swayed by Brian's argument, I am loath to give in and take another leap of faith. I say as much to him.

'There are, as I said, no easy answers. My prayer is that you don't give up now. A life of faith often requires us to walk in darkness believing in a good God and trusting that despite our doubts and evidence to the contrary, He is in control. And as we journey, a deeper understanding helps us be more comfortable with unanswered questions, of living with the see-saw of emotions that vacillate between faith and doubt.'

As Brian is talking I suddenly know what decision to make. I can do no other. I've tried the red pill: other gods, academic achievement, relationships, material things. I know that's not the solution. I'm going to follow this architect of the upside-down kingdom, this loving maverick. I am going to live like he's God, even when I do not understand. And I will believe that he will surprise me with the last chapters of my story.

I feel waves of relief as I tell Brian. Even in my depressed state, hope begins to flicker.

My fervent wish now is for my decision to move from my head to my heart. But there is no going back, only forward, one cat's eye at a time.

10.

STUFFED HEAD SYNDROME

'Thank you,' I say as I look at the audience from the security of the podium. Most people clap, a few more heartily than others. Did the talk go well, I wonder? I still find it hard to judge whether people are genuinely enthusiastic or just being polite.

As the applause subsides, the MC rises to thank me and asks if there are any questions. I always dread this moment. No questions usually means no interest. Fortunately, I see a flutter of raised hands.

'Yes?' I say to the serious-looking woman in the front row. She stands as the mic is passed to her and asks, 'Dr Japhet, how do you know how much of your drama should be story and how much should be message?'

Happy to start with a standard question, I reply: 'If we're doing our job, then you shouldn't be able to differentiate between the story and the message. The story should be the message as it's emotions, not facts, that change us.'

Seemingly satisfied, she sits down and I acknowledge the hand of a hip young man whose face is framed by shoulder-length dreads. 'I've got two questions,' he says. I nod encouragement.

'I've always wondered how you film a rain scene, if it's not raining?'

I laugh. It's one of the filming tricks I love.

'Well, like good South Africans, they make a plan. They send a guy with a hosepipe onto the roof of the house where the scene is being shot. When they need rain, the tap gets switched on.' There is a ripple of laughter.

'So my next question,' the young man says, 'is how do I get to be in your films? It's my dream.'

I'm amazed at how many people aspire to act, deceived by the narrative of glamour, wealth and endless parties. The reality is far from glamorous. Huge amounts of time are spent waiting on set and most actors are dirt poor. So I try my best to dissuade him, but as I know so well, a dream is a powerful thing.

There are a few more questions, which I do my best to answer and then the MC turns to thank me again. Before he can, a middle-aged man tentatively puts up his hand. There is a momentary pause while he waits for the microphone to be passed along to him. He stands. He is tall. Aquiline nose, dark hair receding but still full.

'Thank you for sharing your story,' he begins. 'I've never heard any one talk about "stuffed head syndrome" before.' He hesitates before continuing. 'I presume you meant some form of mental illness because you then proceeded to say that you were "heavily medicated for the protection of the masses". Would I be right?'

I didn't see this coming, but actually I'm glad for the question.

'Yes,' I say, 'you are right. I've suffered from anxiety and depression for most of my life and it's led me into some very dark places. I feel strongly that if a so-called successful person like me doesn't talk about it, I just perpetuate the stigma.' I can feel my cheeks glowing and I begin to speak faster. This often happens when I feel passionate about something. It can be quite off-putting as I can come across as a deranged zealot, but I can do no other. 'For years we've believed the narrative that mentally ill people are crazy or even demon-possessed, so we've locked them up or killed them off. Now, while we don't kill people, we often see them as weak attention seekers who should "just pull themselves together".'

People are looking at me strangely. Where has the calm health professional gone?

'I'm sorry,' I say, 'but that rubbish makes me absolutely mad. Mental illness is as treatable as asthma or diabetes, but because it's the brain we don't see it that way.'

The man puts his hand up again but I can see the MC wants to bring the session to a close, so I say, 'Perhaps we could meet afterwards?' The man looks relieved. I suspect I've touched a nerve.

It's been a long day, and the nervous energy I've expended on the talk has left me drained. I'd rather go straight home, but I have a deep sense that talking to this man is important.

Up close, Jeff, for that is his name, looks like a successful professional. Probably mid-40s, athletic. His blue button-down shirt is tucked into khaki chinos. We find a quiet corner of the conference venue and after ordering some coffee and a slab of chocolate cake (I need the sugar!), we sit down.

'Thank you for your time,' Jeff says. 'I hope you don't mind.'

'Not at all.'

'Telling your story like that was brave.'

'I don't think so. If telling it might help someone, I feel it's both my pleasure and responsibility to do so,' I say.

'How have you managed?' he asks. 'I mean, how do you keep it together? I've been struggling for a while with what you call "stuffed head syndrome" and I don't know that I can carry on.' The pain is evident in his voice.

Despite my desire to normalise this illness, I find myself shocked by my inability to reconcile this seemingly successful man with my perception of what a suicidal person looks like.

'I'm sorry,' I say. I'm not a great listener, I'm too easily distracted, but I know that to be truly present is important, so I try. 'Perhaps you can tell me a little of your story?' I suggest. 'Not your CV. Your story.'

Jeff looks at me warily, like I've asked him to commit a crime. Many people haven't ever thought about their story, let alone shared it and the prospect can be scary. Cautiously he says, 'Okay, I'll try.'

After a halting start he becomes less conscious of my listening and moves back in time, one memory sparking the next. His is what many would term an unremarkable story (although I don't believe there is such a thing) and he is almost apologetic in the telling of it because he does not have a traumatic event to lend credence to his current despair. He has lived the fairy tale. A middle-class upbringing, a loving family. Popular and successful at school and then university. Qualified as a chartered accountant.

Great job, happily married with two children he adores and now, aged 45, he wants to end it all. Why? What possible reason does he have for his despair? For his suicidal thoughts? It's almost as if his pain is worse because he can't find any reason for it. He cannot understand it, but I can: for an analytical person, 90 per cent of the answer is to understand the problem and this is the one thing he can't do.

I find myself caught up in Jeff's story. This invariably happens to me when I listen to other people's stories. To be transported for a short while into a person's world is a privilege.

'When did you start feeling like this?' I ask.

'Probably in the last year,' he tells me. 'It started with me waking up early, like 4am, and then not being able to get back to sleep. I'd lie awake and worry about crazy irrational stuff. What if I get cancer? Then I might lose my job. Then maybe my wife might leave me and take the kids with her and then I would be all alone. And then?' He gives me a wretched look. 'It's the most awful feeling,' he says. 'My heart races, I toss and turn and I can't stop thinking. One worry sparks the next and because there is no answer to any of them, they feed on each other, growing bigger and more out of control, the more I think.'

His story comes pouring out of him. I am sure this is the first time that he's been able to be honest about where he is at and I can sense his relief.

He continues. 'Then morning comes and with it exhaustion, but also some perspective. I am amazed at how illogical my worries seem by the light of day. Then night comes and the cycle repeats itself.' He stops for a minute. 'I became afraid of going to sleep. I began to drink heavily, hoping that it would help, but it only made matters worse.'

He looks at me warily, perhaps to gauge whether I am judging him.

'And now?' I ask in what I hope is my most comforting voice.

'Well, now I'm not just waking early, but I battle to get out of bed in the morning. Not even the daylight helps. I walk around in a fog of deep weariness. It feels like I'm just playing the role that's expected of me. Inside I'm desperate. It's the most terrible feeling imaginable. I can't see a way out.'

I'm finding this hard. Jeff is describing my own symptoms and although, thank God, I have mine under control, his description evokes in me a visceral reaction. Tight chest, pounding heart. I take a few breaths. This is not about me.

'And the worst is that you look absolutely fine,' I say gently.

'Yes,' he says despairingly. 'If someone has a broken leg or some physical illness, people can get their heads around that and empathise. But when I tell people, even my wife, how I'm feeling, they just can't get it. I know what they're thinking: what on earth do I have to be worried about? And they're right. Compared to many, I'm blessed beyond measure. Knowing that I have no reasons for how I'm feeling just makes me feel even more hopeless. Maybe I'm going crazy.' He gives a deep sigh. 'I look into my future and if it weren't for my wife and kids, I think I would end it.'

Jeff looks at me miserably. In situations like these, I'm grateful for my journey.

'Thanks for sharing that with me,' I say. 'If it's any consolation, I understand.'

My sympathy collapses Jeff. He tries futilely to control himself before letting go. He cries in the way that men who have seldom cried do. A deep groaning, his whole body contorting in anguish. I move closer and put my hands on his heaving shoulders. 'It's okay,' I say.

'But what am I going to do?' he says between sobs.

I've had the good fortune of finding wisdom and comfort from people when I needed it most; I pray that I can do the same for him.

'Trust me,' I say firmly. 'You will get better.' I know that when hope dies we die with it, and so the greatest gift I can give him now is hope.

'How can you be so sure?' he says angrily. I know what he's thinking: what right do I have to give him hope when he sees none?

'Because I've been there and come out the other side and I've seen many others do the same,' I say. 'You have bad depression, but it's a treatable physical illness. As physical and treatable as a broken bone.'

Jeff gives me a wry smile. 'I'll take the broken bone,' he says. I smile back.

'Do you think diabetics are crazy?' I ask him.

'No,' he says, puzzled.

'Well, they're not and nor are you. Diabetics, like you, suffer from a chemical imbalance. In their case, it plays havoc with their sugar levels; in yours it sends your moods into a spin.' Jeff is looking a little reassured. 'How do you know that a man is an uncontrolled diabetic?' I ask.

'No idea,' Jeff responds.

'He has flies on his shoes.'

'Huh?'

'Sorry – weak joke told to medical students. The idea being that a diabetic man may dribble some urine on his shoes and because his urine's full of sugar it attracts flies. I told you it was weak.'

Jeff grins, grateful for the interlude. The talk of sugar has refocused me on my chocolate cake, which, without looking, I reach for and send flying. 'Eish, that was dumb,' I say as we both bend down and try to salvage pieces of icing and cake from the floor. 'Unfortunately,' I continue in a more serious tone once we've settled back in our chairs, 'treating depression is not as straightforward as mending a bone. In many ways, our understanding of the brain is still in the Dark Ages. We may know what chemicals are responsible for mood but we are still unsure what makes them play truant. Sometimes it's simple – a traumatic event or a genetic predisposition – but often there is no discernible reason at all.'

Jeff nods as he listens intently.

'The good news is even though the causes are not well understood, there are some highly effective treatments, with more being discovered all the time.'

'So pop a pill and feel good?' he says cynically. 'Not sure about that.

Maybe if I just try to think positive thoughts, get counselling, exercise more, stuff like that … It just freaks me out, the idea of taking pills.'

I try to conceal my frustration. This attitude to taking medication is not uncommon.

'If you got pneumonia now, we could either treat you the same way it's been treated for thousands of years – bed rest and chicken soup; the odds being that after a nasty and lengthy illness you'll get better or die – or we can use antibiotics, shorten the illness and cut down complications. The choice would be yours.' Jeff gives me an awkward smile. 'But medication doesn't work overnight,' I say truthfully. 'It can take a few weeks to feel better. And what works for one person may not work for another. It can be more art than science. The important thing is not to get discouraged, knowing that almost everyone gets better.'

'But it worked for you.' Jeff still looks uncertain. 'How did you know it was working?'

'It was like the sun rose through the fog. I couldn't believe the difference. I could see things in perspective. I felt I could cope with life, enjoy it.'

'And you've been on medication ever since?'

'Thirty years and counting. I was serious when I said that I was "heavily medicated for the protection of the masses".'

'And now?' Jeff asks. 'If you're feeling okay, why don't you stop?'

'Some people have mild depression and they can come off medication, like a diabetic who can control their illness with diet. Others, like me, need it for life.'

I can see that Jeff is struggling to process everything I've said.

'Have you ever asked for help?' I ask him.

'Meaning?'

'A doctor? A psychologist? Or even a pastor?'

He looks at me and takes a deep breath. 'What difference would that have made?

I nod in sympathy. It amazes me that despite the fact that almost one in five people will experience mental illness in their lifetime, it is a topic seldom addressed by the church. 'I know how you feel. I think I lived with depression for years and was too proud or too scared to seek help. It took a crisis to force me to. As you heard me say in my talk earlier, when I did eventually seek help, I went all in: I met with a psychiatrist, a career counsellor and, for good measure, a priest.'

Jeff looks at me deadpan and says, 'So you think I should seek help?' I discern a glimmer of humour – a good sign.

'Yes,' I say. 'And I'll walk this journey with you if you want.'

Jeff nods. 'I can't tell you how just hearing your story and being able to talk to you has made me feel so much better. I'd given up.'

'I know the feeling.'

'Do you mind if I ask you a personal question?' Jeff asks seriously.

'I've just bared my soul in public,' I point out. 'I'm unlikely to mind.'

'Are you sure you don't have diabetes?' he asks.

It's my turn to be nonplussed.

'Because you have a fly on your shoe,' says Jeff.

I really should be more careful when I'm eating chocolate cake.

11.

TAO TIME-OUT

I roll away as black oil floods onto the ground, narrowly missing my head as well as the waiting container. George, our instructor, lets out a deep sigh. 'Lad, when I said, "Gently remove the sump plug," I meant gently.'

'Sorry, George,' I say, as I come out from under the car, 'the damn thing just gave way.'

It's my turn to sigh. Four weeks of 'basic motor car maintenance' classes have not resulted in any tangible improvement in my competency.

'Probably best to let someone else deal with the vehicles when you are out in the mission field,' George says with a tight smile.

Fortunately for any unsuspecting vehicle (or person), I'm not going 'out in the mission field', even though, along with my fiancée and soon-to-be-wife Jayne, I am about to complete my certificate in mission studies at All Nations Christian College. The college, which is a huge rambling red-brick house called Easneye Mansion, was once home to the Buxton missionary family, who played a key role in the Abolition of Slavery Bill. Just outside London, it is surrounded by bluebell woods, narrow hedgerow-lined lanes and grey ploughed fields.

I slowly straighten up. Surely at 34 my body shouldn't hurt so much? But I know that mental pain often manifests physically.

What was I thinking? What was meant to be a time of spiritual and mental 'growth' has been seriously awful. It's also been really hard on our relationship, being engaged in such a monastery-like atmosphere. Once again I feel like my idealism has let me down. First, it was my desire to be a 'saviour' doctor and now it's my discomfort with my 'Sunday' faith. Which does not seem to have progressed much since my blue pill, red pill decision. On the other six days of the week I live a life that is indistinguishable from the secular world and I feel like a fraud.

I again need to make a decision. Either Christ's life and his teachings are true, in which case I need to embrace them with every aspect of my life, including my work, or they're not, in which case I should just chuck the whole thing. Incredibly, my Soul City board and gracious colleagues have allowed me to take 1996 as a sabbatical to explore this question.

Since arriving here, I have become disillusioned. The oppressive grey skies, musty rooms and mustier lecturers have got to me, sending me into a depressive free fall. I had expected that my fellow students would be inspirational, like Eric Liddell, the runner and missionary whose story was made famous by the film *Chariots of Fire*, but, with a few exceptions, my view is that many of the students here are misfits, running away from life.

The question that has consumed me is: What is missing? What will it take for me and others to actually live what we believe? If we were able to do that, perhaps we would change everything.

With only a month left here, my faith has gone backwards. I'm not willing to give it up yet though. Possibly I'm just scared by the nihilist consequences of losing it; but I've already seen and done too much of life to believe that a purely material life will fulfil me.

I shrug off my oil-stained overalls and head out of the barn where the motor mechanics course is held. There are still a few hours before the dreaded weekly meeting with my tutor. I'm sure she's grown as tired of the constant questions I throw at her as I have. A rare watery sun has broken through the monotonous uniformity of the sky, transforming the dull landscape into a palate of russets and rich greens. My spirits lift. It's weird how just the weather can influence my mood.

I decide to use my free time to go for a walk and, for a while, do what I love best – read. So I climb over a wooden stile out of the college grounds and into a field on the adjacent farm. I wander up the gently sloping hill, sidestepping cow dung and tufts of coarse grass. I'm gladdened by the smattering of snowdrops, small, bell-shaped white flowers, that cover the turf, and a welcome herald of spring. But everything in this country looks so ordered, so tame. Even the scents are mild. I miss the drama of Africa.

Towards the crest of the hill I come across an inviting hollow just big enough for me to lie in. The dense bush that hangs over it means that the space is nice and dry too. I take off my jacket and roll it up as a pillow, then settle down with my book. I'm reading the last book in the *Lord of the Rings* trilogy – for the fourth time. I still love it. Tolkien's use of words and imagery is so beautiful. He never ceases to transport me into the world of hobbits, elves and orcs and the quest to save Middle-earth.

Why is it that I keep on coming back to this book, I wonder? Is it just the story, or is it something deeper? It may be fantasy, but the characters are so resonant of life in the real world. The quest is simple: to live for good and to defeat evil. In the same way that Jesus describes a kingdom where the last will be first, it's not the strong who are chosen to lead this quest but the insignificant hobbits. Tolkien peoples his story with characters that mirror the human experience. Some are wholly evil, but most are just struggling to live their better selves. They often fail, but they still have joy, not just happiness; joy is far more satisfying. Every time I read the book, it leaves me wanting to be better than I am, to reach further and dream bigger than is rational.

It starts to drizzle. I move deeper into my hollow in an attempt to keep dry. Looking back down the hill, I can see the dull outline of the college buildings in among the trees. And then, pushing back against the fading winter light, a light comes on in one of the rooms. Soon others follow in a haphazard cascade until the entire building is bathed in a yellow glow. It feels symbolic because I have just had an idea ... a gift from Tolkien, and it is beginning to gather momentum. I wouldn't say 'And then God spoke to me!' because I would not be so sure, but finally I have the exciting sense of a new direction. And with it comes a feeling of relief that this period might not have been a complete waste of time.

My rising excitement is tempered by the awareness of my wet backside. There is no getting away from a persistent English drizzle. I glance at my watch. I walk back down the hill, only this time with more purpose in my stride, to meet with my tutor.

'YOU'RE LOOKING A little brighter, Garth,' Claire Powell greets me as I sink into her sagging office chair. She offers me a mug of tea and a digestive biscuit, the standard fare favoured by all British academics it seems. Claire is a feminist theologian in her mid-40s. She is on a crusade to help people like me see God as a She as well as a He. She is kind and smart, and she has a very English skin nurtured by years of mist and rain. Her usual dress is a neat cardigan and a tweed skirt. 'So what's changed?'

With more enthusiasm than I've been able to muster all year, I begin to tell her about my Tolkien-inspired revelation.

'So this is what I'm thinking,' I say. 'Instead of using story to just deal with health, my plan is to tell stories to inspire people, especially Christians, to live their better selves, to really live the second great commandment, to love our neighbour as ourselves and all that that means.'

Although Claire is listening intently, I'm not sure she's altogether getting it, so I try another way to explain. 'There seems to be so much emphasis on conversion – but what then? When I look around, many of us live lives indistinguishable from the rest of humanity ...' I trail off at this point, realising how lame this sounds. This is not just pie in the sky; it's a whole flipping bakery in the clouds. But Claire smiles encouragingly.

'So you had a mountain top experience,' she says.

'More of a hillock experience,' I say.

'Garth,' she says earnestly, leaning forward, 'you would be joining a long line of Christians who have taught using story, starting with Jesus and his parables and then the Russian authors Dostoyevsky and Tolstoy, and in more recent times Tolkien and CS Lewis.'

I already know the impact of Tolkien on my life, and I have read the whole Narnia series, but I'm intrigued that Claire would bring them up.

'If there is a series of books that I've read nearly as often as I've returned to *Lord of the Rings*, it's the Narnia series. I remember my dad, a secular Jew, telling me how he used to pass CS Lewis on the stairs of his Oxford college and how it was, in part, CS Lewis's writing that led to his conversion.'

'CS Lewis intended the books to be allegorical. In fact, the Narnia series is far more "Christian" than Tolkien's work. Aslan the lion, for instance, is modelled on Jesus.' Claire smiles at the expression on my face. 'You didn't know that?'

I breathe deeply. I am aware that what for months has felt like I have been staring at the jumble of threads on the back of a tapestry has now been turned around, and a picture is emerging.

'Tolkien and Lewis were great friends,' Claire continues, 'and while their works are rich with Christian values, neither of them ever mentions the name of God or Jesus in their works of fiction. I suspect that's what you have in mind – the underlying values?'

For the first time this year I feel really energised. 'That's exactly right!' I say. 'I'm not sure how, or who is going to pay for it, but I want to make a series of socially relevant films that speak to the values shared by all the great faiths. Honesty, compassion, service, perseverance. Even forgiveness.' The faster I talk, the more I can feel my thoughts crystallising. 'Amazing films. Gritty ones about real people who fail and triumph in equal measure. Not the sanitised pie-in-the-sky stuff that so many Christian film makers seem to dish up.'

Claire is generally more comfortable debating the gender of God, but she is gracious.

'And how would people get to see these films?' she asks.

'I think that may be the beauty of the idea,' I say. 'Because they won't be overtly Christian films, they will be able to go onto prime-time TV and big screen cinema, and then later on they could be used in churches, schools, even workplaces.'

I know my tutor wants to support me but I can see I'm losing her. I try a different approach.

'Okay. You know Star Wars?'

'You mean the movies? Yes …' she says, frown lines deepening.

'Well, the creator of Star Wars, George Lucas, believed so much in the power of his films and their characters to lend their popularity to merchandise that he took a cut in his directing fees in order to keep the rights to merchandising. Best decision he ever made. While the Star Wars films have made billions of dollars, the merchandising has made over ten times more. People are willing to pay a premium for a plastic figurine or duvet cover because of the popularity of the films.' If the poor woman was at sea before Star Wars, now she is drowning. I carry on, determined to enthuse her. 'The movies and their stories, the ones I have in mind, will, like the Star Wars films, be just the starting point, the brand builder. It's in the resources that we will develop, the "merchandise" based on the films, for churches, schools and communities that the real transformative power lies. That was the secret of the Soul City success. Think of it as the films ploughing and preparing the field for the seed that is to follow.'

Finally, Claire smiles. It could be the biblical analogy I've just used, but she gets it. This must be one of the strangest tutor sessions she has ever had but I have to hand it to her. She's not afraid to entertain my crazy plan.

'You know, Garth,' she says slowly, 'CS Lewis talks about what he calls "the Tao", a universal sense of morality in all times and cultures that is on the same level of authority as the Bible, because it comes from the Creator. It seems to me that that's what you are talking about, promoting the Tao.'

It is.

Then suddenly Claire asks me: 'Do you know what cats' eyes are?'

'You mean the ones in the road?'

'Yes – the little reflective boxes that show you where the road is in misty conditions.' I nod. I know where this is going! 'A vision like yours, well, I imagine it as a misty road. It's there, but you won't be able to see it all and that's okay. You need only to look for the next cat's eye in the road and follow that, trusting that God has prepared your way in advance.'

I don't tell Claire that I am more than familiar with the cat's eye analogy and that mist and fog have surrounded me for much of my life.

Once again the destination seems clear but the road to reach it not so much.

This time it will take a further nine years for my vision for Heartlines to see the light of day, years that will include many dark nights of the soul, when I will doubt that God is real and, if He is, whether He cares for me, let alone for this vision of mine.

In setting up Heartlines, I would experience the same crisis of relevance that I had had in establishing Soul City, and more profoundly so. Despite personal anecdotes and independent evaluations, which were overwhelmingly positive, I would wonder whether we were actually achieving anything. Or, to quote a phrase, was it just 'flatulence against thunder'? With Soul City we were dealing with tangible issues such as HIV/AIDS and GBV, where the impact was more measurable, but in Heartlines we would be trying to impact on something much more intangible: people's characters, their values and the choices they make.

What sustained me through the fears and uncertainties were the extraordinary people, especially my wife, who travelled alongside me and believed in the vision even when I faltered. While it takes a village to raise a child, it takes a band of believers to birth a vision.

Unlike Soul City, sources of funding for Heartlines were not readily available because we did not fit any Christian or development box. There would be a number of times when we were down to three months of salaries, but so deep was my colleagues' faith in what we were trying to achieve that no one chose to leave. It was humbling.

Years later, I look back at the road that Heartlines has travelled and am struck by how faithfully each cat's eye emerged from the swirling mist on our road just in time – sometimes when we were about to go off course, but more often when we wanted to give up entirely. How like Tolkien's epic tales the battle is seemingly lost but isn't and how unseen are the heroes, the ones behind the scenes who step up and step in.

Incredibly, my Soul City board once again indulges me by agreeing that I may establish a parallel organisation and run both. In 2001, I organise a three-month fellowship in Washington as a base from which to look for seed money to establish the new organisation that came to me when I was on my sabbatical from Soul City. My vision – to tell stories that inspire people to live their better selves, to embrace their true humanity – keeps me going as I criss-cross the United States, having one meeting after another. I meet extraordinary, encouraging people who pepper their responses to me with 'What an amazing idea', 'So needed', 'You must meet—' and the like, but I raise zero money. Nothing.

After five weeks, my vision is on life support. Seven weeks and it has flat-lined. It's dead.

My start-up, fund-raising drive in the United States has come to an end and I am about to return home to South Africa empty-handed.

Then, with one week to go, I am thrown a lifeline.

I have a chance conversation with a young woman at the church we attend.

'I work for World Vision,' she says. 'Have you thought about approaching us?'

Rick Stearns, head of World Vision, has a couple of hours in which he can see me, but after that he is travelling. The trouble is that the meeting is in Seattle and I am in Washington, and now I am stuck in traffic on the way to Dulles Airport. I am already aware that I am going to have to be at my persuasive storytelling best, but also that I need to do it in person. Missing a plane and a crucial meeting is not an auspicious start to a relationship. I'm afraid of heights, but if sky diving was the only option, I swear I would take it, I am that anxious to get to this meeting.

I make it to my departure gate with minutes to spare. Except it's not my gate. I am in the wrong terminal and it will take half an hour to get to the right one. I am going to miss my flight. I can't believe it. I have been so full of hope that this might be my breakthrough, only for it to be dashed in such a dumb fashion. I have seldom felt so gutted. But, hoping against hope, I decide to hot-foot it to the other terminal. Bathed in sweat, I arrive to see a snaking queue at the gate. My flight has been delayed!

I meet with Rick Stearns and secure our first seed money – $15 000.

Heartlines is going to happen.

IN OTHERS' WORDS ...

Knowing that you want to make a change or make a difference – in your personal environment, your community, your country, the world – is all very well, but finding the right vehicle, the strength, the courage to take a step out of what you know and towards something worthy but never very well defined (in my experience, anyway) can be a big leap of faith.

Many people can testify to a feeling of hopelessness or a future that offers you no hope as being one of the most crippling emotional states in which to find yourself. I am one of those people, and in owning, framing and sharing my personal story I have been able to find much strength, even though I still see myself as a work in progress.

Steven Mzee, when looking back to the Nairobi slums of his childhood, where the odds against a bright future were stacked against him, understands an all-consuming feeling of hopelessness. In retrospect, he attributes his escaping a very different and probably much shorter life to God having a plan for him, but it wasn't clear cut. 'I could have taken a wrong turn many times,' he confided during our interview. 'I had no hope in life. But God was keeping an eye on me.'

As a young adult, Steven held the tenuous fraying thread of faith that he could make something of himself. Along the way, certain people stepped in fortuitously to allow him to change a dangerous course or make a better choice in a difficult situation. A turning point came at a particularly dark period. 'I was in my room alone and kind of depressed and I had this discussion with God. I said, "God, today I am going to do one of two things. If I leave this room tonight and walk into church and somebody smiles at me – I am recommitting my life to you."'

Steven got that smile and he felt guided and motivated. His next big leap of faith was deciding to study law, registering with UNISA (not realising it was a distance education university), and travelling to Cape Town to become a student. All his belongings, including his money, were stolen crossing the border into South Africa. In that moment of despair, two Zimbabwean women, strangers to him, paid for his ticket. He discovered that being a foreigner in South Africa had its challenges. He also discovered that his registration at UNISA had not been recorded, and he needed to find a job. He managed to find work as a security guard, which led him to Every Nation Church.

Wanting to find a better life, an education, basic health care and the ability to raise a family in safety and security have been the motivation for millions of people on every continent across the world who risk forging a path or who are forced to flee their homes for one reason or another. Basic human rights as are secured in South Africa's Constitution are, however, far from a given for many people, and personal life circumstances and journeys seldom follow a straight path. Turning point moments are seldom recognised as turning points. Sometimes all we have are the cats' eyes in the mist.

A turning point moment for actor Lillian Dube, whose role as Sister Bettina in Soul City has had such a powerful influence on millions in South Africa, was when her son persuaded her to audition for the series. Being cast in Soul City as a nursing sister suffering from depression came at a time when she herself was struggling with mental health issues and she was able to embrace the role with deep conviction. When she was diagnosed with breast cancer in her 60s, difficult though it was to absorb, she felt that she had been prepared by her Soul City journey to deal with it. It was because of Soul City and the educational role it had played in health care that she was already informed and knew what she needed to do. Her faith and the faith of her friends and followers supported her through treatment and recovery. Her own prayer at a time when prayers were being said for her all over the country was typically generous: 'Please, God,' she prayed, 'show these people that you are a loving God. Let me live.'

Seeing the power of story to make a difference in people's lives, borne out by the popularity of Soul City and the love she continues to be shown to this day, motivated Lillian to take it forward. She became a spokesperson for SADAG (South African Depression and Anxiety Group), speaking out about mental health and normalising its place in the lives of ordinary people; and she became a champion campaigner for cancer awareness.

Lauren Moss is a psychologist who specialises in narrative therapy. She was the middle child in her family, she told me when I went to talk to her about her story. 'I took the role of watching everything going on. I was an observer more than anything. I would observe everyone's stories. When I was young, I wanted to be a photojournalist. That was the first thing I wanted to do. Take photos of people's stories.' It was when she was doing her Master's in Psychology that a light went on. That was when narrative therapy took hold. It also connected with Lauren's other passion, neurology. 'Our brains think in stories,' she explained. 'You go, "Well, this is my story and my story is about my life, where I have lived and my career." If you look at people whose stories are stuck, particularly clients with issues, they keep retelling the same thing. They say things like "I am a victim of my circumstance", "Nothing ever goes right for me". What they are doing is making that neuro path deeper and deeper. I work with them to get them unstuck by rescripting their story.' One technique Lauren uses she calls 'externalising your story', writing it in a different way – using metaphor, for example, or a completely different perspective – can trigger a shift and enable healing to begin. As an example of metaphor she cites the superhero Batman, the caped crusader who fights crime and effects justice, after suffering a traumatic event in childhood. 'When you say "Batman", people go, "Oh, yes. I can relate to that."'

Jonathan Shapiro was a child who had nightmares, and it was his mother who encouraged him to draw them, taking ownership of the fearsome creatures in his dreams, thereby changing the narrative. Using monster as metaphor continued to be a technique he would hone and develop in his career as a cartoonist.

Underpinning all of Brent Lindeque's 'making a difference' ventures is the desire to turn fear into hope, with the vehicle being telling a story in one form or another, via different media and platforms. Often driven only by a strong belief that something radical might be effective and that a narrative is at the heart of it, his instinct has proved sound. 'Look for the heroes,' is his advice. 'In times of tragedy, there will always be heroes.'

Pastor Leigh Robinson has personal experience of deep tragedy. He grew up in Durban, in a home with an emotionally absent father who was an alcoholic and who brought pain to the family, and especially to his mother for some years through an extramarital affair. Leigh moved to Canada to pursue his theological studies. It was here that he met his first wife, Esther, and they had a son, Jonathan. When Jonathan was two years old, on a family visit to South Africa, Esther and Leigh's sister Jayne were involved in a head-on collision. Both were killed instantly. Consumed with grief, Leigh returned to Canada with his two-year-old son.

'And in God's providence He led me and Irene together,' Leigh recounted. 'We got married about 14 months after Esther died, which pragmatically was the right time. Jonathan needed a mother, and I needed a wife, and the school year was about to start, and if we didn't get married then we would have had to wait another year. And we were certain that God had led us together, we were not in doubt of that.' It soon became clear, however, to both Irene and Leigh, that remarriage was emotionally too soon for Leigh. 'The result of that was that our first few years of marriage were really turbulent,' they both admitted.

It didn't help matters when they moved to South Africa, where Leigh became the pastor at Durban North Baptist Church. This required Irene making another huge leap of faith. Leigh acknowledges her courage and the sacrifices she made. 'She left behind her family, her friends, her country, her culture, her support system,' he said. 'She was married to a man who didn't yet love her, and she had a son who she hadn't given birth to. And so I think we both thought we had died and gone to hell. And on top of that I was the pastor and she was a pastor's wife, and pastors and wives are not supposed to have problems.'

Leigh could not have known it at the time, but in retrospect, he said, 'My loss of Esther and the lessons I learned through that equipped me for the next 40-plus years of pastoral ministry in ways that I never could have imagined, because I spent my years dealing with people who were grieving one kind of loss or another. One of the major contributions that I've made to the lives of people in our congregations has been journeying with them through their grief.'

As a pastoral couple, counselling other couples through difficult marriages became something the Robinsons were well equipped to do. In being open and honest about their own marital struggles, allowing themselves to be vulnerable and sharing their journey candidly with their congregation, in turn gave others a safe space to share their stories. 'Because we've been vulnerable, they know that they're not going to be judged,' said Leigh. 'So they feel safe to share, because they know they're not talking to two perfect people, but two fellow strugglers.'

Many of those I interviewed spoke about a spiritual intervention or a word of guidance or wisdom from an unexpected source at a time of uncertainty or darkness.

For Seth Naicker, one such person was his Afrikaans teacher at school, Dawn Naidoo. He struggled with the subject and was in danger of jeopardising his further education if he failed it. 'She said, "Seth, I'm really not too interested in how well you do in Afrikaans, I just need you to pass. But I'm more interested in what I'm teaching you for your values, for your life.' Another time, when he was in matric he lost a friend, Terrance, through gang violence. Terrance died of a gunshot wound to the head, and anger and thoughts of vengeance were on his friends' minds. It was Terrance's mother, grieving the loss of her son, who asked them not to act in anger.

'His mother told us that she didn't want us to create any reaction or rebuttal or find a way to get back at the guys who did this. She told us we needed to leave it to the law, and that God would be in control. I struggled with it. There's definitely a time when you feel I want real vengeance. Our friend died, and we've got to do what we need to do to get people back. But her words kind of spoke, and we did a thing that young boys did not do back then. We cried. But it created a very deep community. I'm still in contact with a lot of those friends today.'

Alison Harris has a deep Christian faith. In our interview she described a visceral feeling when she felt God was guiding her in a certain direction. 'Part of what I have realised is that with listening, it is not just an audible listen. It is also listening to those nudges inside, which I believe is God. I went through a stage in my life where I thought I was absolutely crazy because I would walk past people and go from happy to bursting into tears and feeling this incredible sorrow. I did not know where it came from. I remember a specific feeling in the tips of my fingers where I just felt an emotion. I spoke to my dad about it. I went to him thinking he was going to tell me there was something wrong with me and he just said, "Well, me too." It was amazing that we started to connect over that. I believe that God instilled in us things that prompt us. My dad challenged me to listen to it rather than be overwhelmed by it. Then it would happen and I would just look around and there would be a person crying in that moment and I just started practising going over and chatting to them.'

Irene Robinson remembered a dark period when she was 18, a young woman, alone, trying to discern even the glimmer of a cat's eye in Calgary. 'It was the year I remember watching Martin Luther King and Bobby Kennedy assassinated on TV, and just crying my eyes out. I mean, I don't even know them, but I think because I was so sad inside, this trauma that I was watching on the news, I just cried and cried and cried. Anyways, I just got more and more depressed and lonely. I didn't know anybody, I didn't have a life, trying to find a job that's going to make me happy, and working for this lady who also was unhappy. And then I started thinking, if there's any answers to these questions, maybe they're in the Bible. So I went to look in her bookcase, and sure enough I found a Bible, and I started reading from Matthew, and it was like water to a thirsty soul. I got to Chapter 7, verses 13 and 14 where it says, "Wide is the gate that leads to destruction and there are many going that way, but narrow is the gate that leads to life and few will find it." And it was as if God said to me, "There is another way, Irene, than what you know. Just keep looking."'

Motivational speaker Quinton Pretorius is another person who believes that at significant and painful moments along his life's path there has been a quiet, comforting intervention. 'My faith has been key in terms of where I find myself. The cornerstone of my relationship with Christ has been a motivator. It is more than a motivator – it is central to where I find myself. There have been many experiences where I feel like Christ has shown up in powerful ways.' He described one such incidence – what I call a 'God-incidence' – during a stressful period as a teenager. 'My youth pastor was picking us up for the evening service and as the kombi was leaving our house, I remember my mother and stepfather were having a huge fight. Throwing furniture at each other and it was just a disaster.

'A couple of weeks prior to that, I saw one of my youth pastors hug his daughter. I sat there and I thought to myself, I am sixteen and I have never been hugged by a man in my life before. What I saw my youth pastor do to his daughter was something new. I did not know what that felt like. When we got to church, my pastor did not say anything. He took me to the back of the church hall and he just hugged me. It was like God himself came out of heaven and hugged me.'

Over and over again, in different ways and in different surroundings, the stories of interventions that were told to me by the amazing range of people I interviewed – personal, intimate, vividly real or quite invisible, many of them seemingly random – kept bringing me back to that point of stillness, where listening and hearing can be life-changing, not only for others but for oneself. Being privileged to share such experiences with fellow travellers creates a connection, if only to feel that we are not alone.

PART 4

INFLUENCING – THE POWER OF STORY
TO CHALLENGE THINKING AND CHANGE
BEHAVIOUR

Some years back I had lunch with a director in Hollywood and in one powerful sentence he summed up the pervasive power of story to shape our values and influence our behaviour. He said, 'America is today what Hollywood portrayed it to be 20 years ago', namely, the mores and values portrayed by a small group of creatives in their stories became normative for society; art leading culture rather than art reflecting culture.

And people are increasingly recognising this power. When Steve Denning, ex-head of talent management at the World Bank, was asked why use story in business, he replied, 'Simple, nothing else works.' He went on to say, 'When it comes to inspiring people to embrace a vision or a change in behaviour, storytelling isn't just better than the other tools. It's the only thing that works.' And work it does.

People in marketing have been embracing story power for years. They realised early on that the best advertisements were mini-stories. The number of books, TED talks and consultants preaching story as a key business tool these days seems to be rising exponentially. Want to market powerfully? Build it around a story. Want to motivate your team with your vision? Tell them a story. Want to do a memorable talk? Start with a story.

It's strange that a human behaviour as old as we are is being 'discovered' as the hot new thing.

Scientists in Paul Zak's lab at Claremont Graduate University discovered that oxytocin, a hormone secreted by the brain, is key to the signal 'it's safe to approach others'. We produce it when we are trusted or shown a kindness and it motivates us to co-operate with others. Good for business! They decided to see whether they could 'hack' the production of oxytocin by exposing groups of people to different stories and then measuring their oxytocin levels. They found that stories that managed to capture their attention and transport them into the character's world led to spikes in oxytocin. One group of people watched a short story narrated by the father of a boy dying of cancer. Their oxytocin levels shot up and many donated their participation fees to a children's cancer charity. A similar but less engaging narrative led to no increase in oxytocin and people hanging onto their participation fee.

Zak is also the scientist who has extensively researched the 'hero's journey' impact in story. I know that many of the stories that have had a powerful influence on me have followed that format. The Jungle Doctor books, Tolkien's *The Lord of the Rings* and the Narnia series by CS Lewis probably resulted in my brain being awash in oxytocin.

Interestingly, science has begun to uncover some really amazing things about what's happening in your brain when you are exposed to a great story. In 2006, researchers in Spain discovered that when we are presented with vivid stories, more than just the small language centre of our brains light up. They found that lots of different centres light up, depending on what is in the story. If a ballet scene is beautifully described in a novel, for example, the sight and movement centres of our brains light up (even those of us who think they can't dance!); we don't have to see the ballet being performed on a stage or on a screen. Similarly, when a smell such as the beautiful scent of jasmine is described in prose, our smell centre lights up. In short, we can have an emotional, whole-brain sensory experience rather than the tiny blip that happens when we are exposed to fact. And because we are far more emotional beings than rational beings, it's not surprising that emotive stories have the power to influence our decision-making and behaviour.

Not only do great stories, fact or fiction, light up our neurons like Christmas trees, they also have a profound effect on our brain's chemistry. Our response to stories, true or not, dished up via screens, the printed page, or audio, can illicit the same stream of hormones as if we were going through the events ourselves. Cortisol is the hormone produced by our bodies in response to stress or danger. Dopamine is our brain's 'feel good' drug, produced in anticipation of, or as a result of, a pleasurable event. It's thanks to dopamine that we binge-watch a TV series.

As Paul Zak has shown, the wonder drug of storytelling, however, is: oxytocin. When you listen, really listen, to someone's story your brain produces oxytocin. It is those molecules that transport you into their world, enabling you to understand and empathise with them. As I will recount in this section, Part 4, the final part of this book, the practice of sharing our personal stories at Heartlines has had us awash in oxytocin, transforming our relationships.

Many of those I interviewed for this book told personal stories of seemingly insurmountable odds standing in the way of their goals, obstacles there seemed no way around, and yet – through the power of a story shared – a door opened, a hardened attitude shifted, funding for a project was raised, and lives were changed for the better as a result.

Oxytocin is the generosity molecule, the peace drug.

I am planning to put it into the world's water supply. This may take a while, but reading this book should have shown you by now that I'm not one to be daunted by what might seem like a crazy, unrealistic vision ...

12.

STORY AS DIAGNOSIS, STORY AS TREATMENT

'What's this? What's this?' Thabang roars, spittle flying from his mouth as he shoves a paper in his wife Matlakala's face. Grabbing her by the neck, he flings her to the floor. 'A protection order? You think that's going to stop me?!'

His young son cries out and grabs him by the leg. 'Daddy, please stop, you're hurting Mom.'

A bull of a man, Thabang swats his son away and advances on his mother. With a sickening rhythm, he proceeds to kick her.

'Stop, stop!" she screams as she covers her head and rolls away, gesturing frantically to her children to hide.

'I'll kill you before any protection order saves you! Do you hear me?' Thabang begins tearing up the piece of paper, his wife's limp form curled into a ball at his feet.

And then he stops, listens. From outside in the street comes a wave of sound. It crashes into the front room as if a hundred demented drummers have been let loose outside the house. Thabang rushes to the front door and flings it open. He is greeted by an extraordinary sight and the sound is deafening. His neighbours from all sides are standing across the street and they are not smiling. They have a variety of cooking pots and spoons in their hands and they are banging them with vigour and fierce emotion.

'Enough is enough!' they shout.

Thabang is astonished. He raises his voice, trying to be heard above the clamour. 'But … but she's my wife …' he says.

'Enough is enough!' they shout back.

A police car hurtles into view and the credits roll.

'SHEREEN! HAVE YOU seen this?' I hold up a press clipping from the *Cape Times* – 'Women Protest against Domestic Abuse in Khayelitsha'. 'This is as a result of the series, right?'

It's uncanny. It feels like they've screen-grabbed the pot-banging scene and pasted it onto this article.

Shereen smiles at me over her morning cup of coffee. 'No question,' she says. 'We picked up the idea from some work in South America while we were in the research phase for this gender-based violence series. There was no record of anything similar in South Africa, but it comes out of a community coming together and practical but innovative ways to help each other. Hence the preceding scene in the community hall.'

The scene Shereen is referring to is a powerful one in itself.

The community in which the Sereti family lived was a close and supportive one, where people knew each other and helped each other. Except when it came to husband and wife issues; domestic problems – that was a private affair. But a few months back a man had killed his partner and the community had seen it coming. Despite the woman's pleas for help, no one wanted to get involved. 'Too dangerous' was the common refrain; 'It's their business' was another. But then she was dead and who knew whose daughter, sister or friend might be next?

A community meeting was called and a police representative was invited. A heated debate ensued. The police were blamed, men were blamed, the government was blamed, people got emotional. There was no solution in sight.

Then a strange thing happened. A young man stood up and said: 'What if we let the man know that we know that he is an abuser? That we are not prepared to sit back and let it happen?'

'And get killed?' people shouted.

'No,' he said calmly. 'We make a noise, a huge noise, outside the house, so that he knows that what he is doing in "private" is public.'

'And then you call us,' the policeman interjected, relieved for once to not be the focus of the community's ire.

'Yes, then we call you guys,' the young man said.

'But how would the abuser hear us?' someone called out. 'There is always shouting in the streets. How would shouting help?'

A woman in the middle of the hall stood up. 'What about pots?' she said. 'We all have metal pots and spoons. If enough of us bang pots, there is no way he won't hear us.'

I THINK BACK to the day in Alex, a lifetime ago now, it seems, when Shereen Usdin appeared in the cubicle in between patients and announced that she was coming to help me with Soul City. A lot of years have passed since then. None of them have been what you might call plain sailing, and yet here we are, eleven years on.

The Houghton house that is Soul City's offices is a lovely space. Huge rooms, pressed steel ceilings. Set in a large garden dominated by a fenced pool and an ancient avo tree. This morning the parquet floors are golden, illuminated by the morning sun streaming through the glass doors of the sitting room. Sadly, however, what seemed perfect when we were five is impractical now that we are fifteen and growing rapidly. Soon we are going to move to offices and officially 'grow up'.

'We're getting reports all the time of this taking off.' Shereen brings me back to the present and the GBV series that has made such an impact around the country.

It never fails to amaze me – the reach and influence of story.

'The helplines have been crazy,' Shereen goes on. 'At last count they'd had over 120 000 calls.'

'Credit to you. You made this happen,' I say and I mean it.

We sit in companionable silence, each lost in our own thoughts.

The team, of course, is no longer just Shereen and me. Research has been central to our being able consistently to deliver a show that is both relevant in content and compelling in storyline. An early challenge revolved around the audience-centred research process we were using to ensure that we were developing a series that would both entertain and also resonate with our audience's lives. This had led to some fearsome showdowns with the creative team.

I remember one in particular where director Bobby Heaney and writer Richard Beynon had screamed at us in unison.

'What do you mean you want to get rid of this scene? It's the high point of the series!'

We tried to explain that while they might love the scene in which a woman's ancestors had instructed her on how to breastfeed, our research showed that the audience would think she was being cursed.

Shereen and I, too, have had our fair share of passionate disagreements. Once, over lunch, we had such a shouting match that the restaurant told us that either the other patrons would need to leave or we would and that they favoured the latter.

I stand up to get us a coffee refill. When I come back to the table, I tell Shereen that I need her help.

'You always do,' she says. 'I think we've established that.'

'No, this is serious. I know I can persuade people to part with their money—'

'You can and do.'

'And I have an ability to talk with confidence on subjects I know little about—'

'That's also true.'

'But I often stumble when I try to explain what we do. Take last night, for example. I met this potential funder, told him about what we do, that people love our TV series, our radio dramas and glossy booklets and that we have proven impact. "So you're like an ad agency," he said. I tried to explain that we are very different, but I just wasn't getting through. All I got was a repeat. "So you're like an ad agency." I wanted to scream. Needless to say no bucks from him.'

'Frustrating,' Shereen responds sympathetically.

'Hugely,' I say. 'I feel like I'm losing funding because I'm meant to be an expert communicator and I'm not doing a good job of communicating our communication!'

'You're not that bad,' she says with mock seriousness. 'The way I approach those conversations, if it will help, is by equating what we do to the difference between a Rolex watch and a forgery.'

Huh? Shereen is not a watch person.

'Well, superficially they're both Rolexes,' Shereen says. 'They look identical, but take a deeper look and you'll see that one is the product of years of research, investment and expertise and the other is not.'

'Morning!' Sue Goldstein interrupts us as she walks into the sun-drenched room, coffee in hand, and settles onto the couch next to Shereen. 'What are we talking about?'

A phrase comes into my mind: a three-stranded cord is not easily broken. My biblical knowledge is not great but I remember that verse. How fortunate I have been to work with these two people. I was a lone nut. Then Shereen joined me and I was nut no more. And then there was Sue. Sue is a doctor who has specialised in health promotion. When Sue joined Soul City ... we became rope. I catch my thoughts as they cartwheel off at a tangent.

'Watches,' I say. 'You'll catch up.' I turn back to Shereen. 'So how do you explain that we are more genuine Rolex than fake?'

Sue looks baffled so I take pity on her.

'I was asking Shereen to explain the complexity that goes into developing a series like this one. On GBV.'

'Okay ... but where do watches come in?' Sue asks, still perplexed.

Shereen explains, 'I was using a real versus forgery analogy to break it down for Garth. Superficially, they might look the same but they aren't. Our dramas and publications may look the same as others that are produced, but they aren't. Because of our research process.'

'Ah,' says Sue.

'Go on,' I say. I'm beginning to like this analogy.

'The critical thing is to get people to understand why we spend so much time and money on research before we produce anything. People assume, incorrectly, that if information is repeated often enough, billboards, radio and TV ads and so on, people will get it and make the right choices. Information is a starting point but it's not enough. We need to find out why we behave the way we do.'

'Decades of smoking education have proved how wrong that approach is,' Sue chips in, 'information repeated, supposedly hammered home.' Sue is an anti-smoking zealot. 'Large text on the boxes – SMOKING KILLS. Gory pictures of blackened lungs. Teenagers laugh at that stuff. Research showed that most young people are much more interested in the opposite sex than dying sometime in the future. So messages like "Do you want to taste like an ashtray?" were developed.'

'Gross!'

'Precisely.'

'And that worked?'

'Partially. But what was also discovered was that people would stop smoking if it became too expensive or too difficult. That's what has really brought smoking levels down: price and bans on smoking in public places.'

'It's frustrating,' Shereen interjects. 'Everyone knows that information alone is not enough, that you have to get out there and ask people questions, understand the environment, what are the enablers or obstacles to the desired behaviour, stuff like that. We already know this. And yet every time we tackle a new public health issue, we repeat the same mistakes.'

Years later, in the midst of the COVID-19 epidemic, that will be exactly what happens.

'Okay,' I say, 'then how would you explain to a layman how we approach GBV?'

'Person,' says Sue. She hasn't given up on me.

'Person,' I respond.

169

'Well, I like to use the analogy of medical diagnosis and treatment,' Sue says. 'Our medical training has drummed into us the importance of getting the full story, doing an examination, and only then making your diagnosis, not before. If your diagnosis is based on assumptions, then your treatment will likely fail. It's the same with GBV. We can't just assume we know what causes it and rush into solutions. Like splashing the slogan "Real Men Don't Beat Women" everywhere and thinking it's going to change behaviour. Wrong diagnosis, wrong treatment.' Sue is vehement. 'Drives me mental!' she adds.

'Because we wanted to make a meaningful intervention,' says Shereen, taking over and getting back to Soul City and the episode we've been discussing, 'we needed to ask questions. Like why does a woman stay in a relationship if she's being physically or emotionally abused? And what causes men to be abusers?'

I think how foreign the concept is to me. I thank God for my dad.

'We've found that it's certainly not lack of information,' Shereen continues. 'Often it's what she believes about herself. Things like, "I must have done something to deserve it." Or it's simply that she doesn't believe she has any power to make choices. If it's not that, then it's often that she believes bearing the abuse silently is the norm in her community. What happens between partners is seen as a private affair, so standing up and making a fuss is frowned upon.'

'So if I think that people around me accept a behaviour as normal, I'm likely to believe it is too, even if I know it's wrong?'

'Absolutely,' Sue interjects. 'It's often the answer to why some men are abusers. They grew up watching their mum get pummelled by their dad so they're likely to think it's okay. Even if a poster on every telephone pole says it's wrong, they still might end up doing the same to their partner as their dad did to his.'

'What really makes me mad,' says Shereen, 'is that it's often the system that lets women down. We've heard so many stories of women, after having plucked up the courage to report the bastard to the police, getting turned away because either the police couldn't care or they just don't know what to do.'

The more we talk the more emotive this becomes for us. This must be how it is for all women, I know, but for me it feeds into a deep-seated hatred for any oppression of the weak by the strong. I'm grateful that at Soul City we did not rush into thinking we knew the answers, but have taken time to understand this issue. As a result our 'treatment', like the problem, has been complex and multi-faceted.

At its heart has been story. Intuitively, I knew that story had the power to change us, but it was only in later years that I discovered the supporting science: the insights that have allowed us to use story more like a skilled surgeon uses a blade than an amateur butcher.

'It's so lekker after the hard yards you've put in the last two years that you get to see the effects,' I say to Shereen, for she has worked tirelessly on developing the GBV-themed series, 'especially when we've had so much pressure to just DO something.'

'Ah thanks, you're so sweet ... sometimes.'

I let the 'sometimes' go – this time. It feels so good hearing how Matlakala, the woman in the series who is suffering physical abuse at the hands of her intimate partner, has given other women courage. We took her on a journey. She realises she can make a change. And she has inspired others to believe they can make a change too.

'I find it so interesting,' I say. 'Women talk about Matlakala as if she was real.'

'She is as real to them as we are to each other,' says Shereen. 'There's a term for it: parasocial interaction. When you develop a close personal relationship with a character, or characters, in a series like ours. The screen fades away and you see yourself. You identify with the characters as if they were close friends. As a result, the influence on your life can be as, if not more, dramatic as the stories that play out on the screen.'

'Reminds me of The Archers story. Do you guys know it?' I ask.

'Vaguely,' Sue says.

'It's an extraordinary story. The Archers is a radio drama series in the UK. In fact, it is the longest-running radio drama in history. It's still running today. In the 50s, it was wildly popular, so much so that three out of five British adults listened on a regular basis. In 1955 one of the most popular characters died in a fire. What happened next was quite extraordinary. Newspapers ran banner headlines: "Grace Archer Dies in Fire". The UK went into mourning. People wanted to lay wreaths and attend her funeral. She was a fictional character, yet people suspended rationality. Not only did they believe she was real, but they felt they had a relationship with her.'

As I talk I am aware that I am talking about myself. It's not that strange. The jungle doctor and characters in other stories since have been very real to me.

'Help! He's killing me! Stop him! Help! Please help me—'

Strangled screams come from the garden.

Our tranquillity shattered, we scramble from our seats and rush outside

'I'll teach you to –' thump! '– steal tools from my shed –' thump! '– you thief!'

Our eyes take in the bizarre scene. Baba Victor, our 70-year-old gardener, who barely tops five feet, has a terrified young man in a headlock, punctuating his furious words with surprisingly effective punches. Colleagues Thuli and Joel are trying to free the hapless chancer from the old man's grasp, but Victor hangs on grimly. It is only when his false teeth are dislodged that the victim is able to struggle free.

'Call the police!' Joel shouts. He is holding the young man with one hand while keeping Baba Victor at bay with the other.

'Yes, please! Call the police!' begs the young man.

The rest of the Soul City team floods out into the garden. Much as we all abhor violence, most of us can't stop ourselves from laughing. The sight of the revenge of the geriatric trumps our best intentions.

What a wonderful mixture we are. Thuli, whom we met first while working in Alex Clinic, leads our community research, the heart of our work, with sensitivity and insight. Moeresi, our regal administrator, who always seem to be calm in the midst of our chaos. Joel, whom I met when I was setting up a Saturday school in Alex, is a young man who came back from the brink of crime to lead some of our community work. And there is Sally – the young adult educator who is responsible for our booklets, of which we print a million at a time. And all the others … We are a passionate and eclectic mix.

'So,' I say to Sue and Shereen as we amble back indoors, 'is there a name for that?'

'For what?' asks Shereen.

'Geriatric violence against youth.'

Silence. They look at me quizzically.

'Justice,' I say with mock seriousness. 'But hypothetically it was wrong,' I add in the same tone. 'We, the Soul City community, stood by and let it happen.' I'm stirring. I know I'll get a reaction and I do.

'Oh, come off it, Garth! You know this is different!' Shereen says, not sure whether I'm being serious. 'The tables were turned, the weak rose up against the strong. Unlike what happens to most women. Communities know they're being abused and do nothing and we know why. "It's a private affair." Such a bloody cop-out, I don't buy that. But I do understand the fear, and I'm not sure I would want to take on a raging man full of drink and anger. Which is why we crafted this story to show another way. We portray the community deciding to stand up, to organise. They decide that a man beating up a woman is not "normal behaviour" and we give them a way to confront the man through banging pots. And those stories get people thinking because for them Soul City is their community. Actually, it's mind-blowing. The fictitious world we have created in Soul City, because of parasocial interaction, is real to them. And because they love and respect our characters, those characters' influence can be even greater than the influence of real people. Do you have any idea how many communities have actually named themselves "Soul City"?'

I draw a blank on this. I shake my head.

'At least twelve and counting,' says Shereen. 'And poor Lillian Dube! People really can't get enough of her. They absolutely refuse to believe that she is not Sister Bettina from Soul City.' We both chuckle at this; we know only too well how believable the actor is. 'Remember the community event we did, when that government official was speaking about HIV/AIDS?'

I remembered it well. It was quite embarrassing. No one was interested in listening to the official and they showed it, but when 'Sister Bettina' spoke it was a completely different story. It's the same today. She is mobbed wherever she goes.

'The same thing happened with Soul Buddyz,' says Shereen, referring to our children's series. 'Because we showed a group of kids getting together and taking on community challenges in the story, we inspired kids to want to be just like them.'

'I still remember the hundreds of letters we received during the first series, kids desperate to be Buddyz,' I say. 'That's when we decided to set up Buddyz clubs in schools. How many Buddyz clubs do we have now?' I'm ashamed that I don't have the number at my fingertips.

'Seven thousand and counting,' says Sue with a big smile. She has been the driving force for the development and success of Buddyz.

The Buddyz series was another idea I had had that was inspired by story. When I was young, I devoured the Enid Blyton Famous Five and Secret Seven series. I wanted to be just like those kids. I gathered a group of friends, built a fort, developed a secret handshake, passports, everything. I had it all mapped out. But my 'gang' was less keen so it faded. Until I resurrected it in Soul Buddyz.

How fortunate I am, I think to myself. So few people get to live their dream and to do it with people they like and respect. I've been inspired by story and now I get to tell stories that inspire.

'Better get to work,' Shereen says as we walk back into the 'sitting room'.

'Likewise,' Sue says.

I bid them both goodbye as I make my way down the passage to the toilet, now converted into my 'office', which, as my colleagues have pointed out with glee more than a few times, is an appropriate place for me to be.

13.

PITCH AND PERSUASION

Laughing with delight but quite out of control, I zigzag crazily down the toboggan run, faster and faster. Snow-laden pines flash past. In desperation I try jamming my heels into the snow to bring my descent to a halt but it doesn't work. What does is an icy bank and a bone-shaking thump, which ejects me from the seat and sends me sliding in a tangle of limbs. Thankfully, the bank also stopped me from being catapulted into the void and becoming tomorrow's headlines – certainly not the headlines I am hoping for.

'You've done this before?' a hotel guest had asked me with a mildly puzzled frown when I announced my snap decision to sledge down to the conference centre in the valley below.

I hadn't, but how hard could it be? Wearing a cloak of bravado over my business attire, I'd set off confidently.

Now that I think about it, perhaps it wasn't the wisest idea. Still laughing, I do a quick check. Nothing broken, but I'm a complete mess, snow everywhere, more snowy brambles in my hair than Bilbo Baggins. Shaken but exultant, I decide my tobogganing career is at an end and I walk the rest of the way into Davos. I might look like I've just lost a fight with a polar bear, but my next encounter is going to be a different kind of challenge. I have a meeting with Richard Branson, a meeting that could change everything.

Davos, in picture-postcard Switzerland, is a fairy-tale setting for this annual get together of the world's political and economic heavyweights, and quite a leap from the dusty, litter-strewn streets of Alexandra township in South Africa where Soul City began. The journey that has taken me from there to here has certainly not been as smooth-sailing as my ill-considered toboggan ride just proved to be, but I'm here nevertheless.

I brush myself down and approach the main entrance to the World Economic Forum. I flash the badge that bestows rights to the inner sanctum. I pass through metal detectors under the stern gaze of the Swiss police.

As a so-called social entrepreneur and Schwab fellow of the World Economic Forum, this is my fourth visit to Davos. Even so, I feel like a steak at a vegan restaurant. Almost all the other delegates own a country or at least are worth a zillion dollars and they're here either to purchase another country or to increase their net worth. Nothing makes this clearer than what I call 'the Davos jerk': people walk around looking at badges, not faces. If your badge says King, President or the like, the head jerks up; if not, they avoid eye contact and move on. Needless to say, not many people look up at me.

There are, however, some great opportunities and my meeting with Branson is one of them. I arrive at the meeting room and Pamela Hartigan, the bundle of energy who heads up the Schwab Foundation, greets me. 'Just waiting for Richard,' she says. 'He should be here shortly.'

Seated next to Pamela is Isaac Durojaiye, a fellow social entrepreneur, from Nigeria. 'Hey, Garth!' he bellows. 'This will be good, ja?' Isaac is a giant of a man, over seven feet tall. Before he set up his DMT Mobile Toilets, Nigeria, he was the President's bodyguard. He describes DMT as renting out mobile toilets to 'widows and orphans' in informal settlements who then operate them as a business, providing employment and sanitation in one. 'It's a shit business but a good one,' he laughs.

Richard Branson, instantly recognisable with his shaggy blond mane, walks in. He greets us warmly before sitting down. Pamela asks me to begin by introducing Soul City and myself, so I launch into my pitch of how over the last twelve years we've used story through TV and radio dramas to deal with key health issues such as HIV/AIDS.

Looking slightly bored, Branson says, 'So you've produced a few films?'

'Er ...' I stammer. 'We actually have one of the most watched and listened to programmes on TV and radio.'

'Very nice. So people like what you do?' Branson asks while looking at a point above my head.

'They love Soul City!' I say. 'It reaches over 45 million people in ten countries. It's as well known among black South Africans as Coca-Cola.'

'And probably better for you,' Branson says with a half-smile.

'Much,' I say. 'Rather like George Lucas did with the merchandise that came out of the Star Wars movies, we leverage the popularity of our brand, stories and characters to further influence hearts and minds. Our 35 million publications are based on the stories and characters from Soul City.'

Pamela interjects helpfully. 'Tell Richard the story about the actor, Garth. I think it's a great illustration of how powerful your model is.'

'Well, we've got this actor who plays a nurse called Sister Bettina. It's amazing. Even though people know she's an actor, she's constantly called upon to give medical advice. She draws huge crowds wherever she goes. It's incredible.'

Branson laughs. 'How about selling her to us?' he suggests. 'We could set up Virgin Family Planning – I like the sound of that!'

Pamela and I laugh politely.

'Very impressive,' Branson says. 'And your impact?'

'Perhaps the most compelling evidence came from a large study in 2005,' I tell him, 'which indicated that Soul City was a major reason for preventing half a million new HIV infections.' I pause to let that sink in, then quickly continue. 'Let me give you a personal example. I was recently pulled over for speeding and was resigned to a hefty fine. When I said I worked for Soul City, the cop said, "You mean like on TV?" "Yes," I replied. "No, man, then how can I fine you?" the cop said. And then he spontaneously launched into the story of how the storyline about diarrhoea had saved his child's life.' I stop. Every word I'm saying is true. 'We have thousands of stories like that,' I add.

'Wonderful,' Branson says distractedly.

I can sense with an instinct honed by years of rejections that while Richard Branson gets what we do, it isn't for him. He turns to Isaac and invites him to describe his business. Isaac happily obliges with a colourful description of DMT, Nigeria.

Branson is immediately intrigued. 'If I wanted to brand your toilets, how much would that cost?' he asks.

'With your Virgin brand?' Isaac responds quizzically.

'No. I want to put British Airways branding all over them!' Brandon laughs and Isaac's face breaks into a broad grin.

'$100 per toilet!' he says promptly.

'Deal!' Branson replies. 'I'll take a hundred!'

I leave the meeting despondent. If an out-of-the-box thinker like Richard Branson doesn't get excited about Soul City, then who will? Life was a lot simpler sewing up a wound or setting a fracture. People got that.

Pamela has followed me out. 'Come, let's grab a coffee,' she says. Across the table she is sympathetic. 'I understand the significance of your work, Garth, and I thought Richard would too. Perhaps we'll have better luck with the head of the Gates Foundation.'

'Perhaps,' I say, without conviction. 'But' – I grin at a sudden memory – 'this was way better than the time I met the Queen and Prince Philip ...'

'Really?' Pamela looks dubious.

'Yes, really. I met them in 1995, shortly after we launched the first series of Soul City on maternal and child health. They asked me what we did and when I told them, Prince Philip said to me, "Why bother? They're going to die anyway!"'

'I've heard he's like that,' Pamela says when she finally gets her laughter under control. She grasps my hands in hers. 'Don't get down, Garth,' she says earnestly. 'What you are doing is important but it's not instant. Most people don't get that. Complex problems, especially those that involve human behaviour, will take years of hard work to influence. Most funders want quick results.'

'So British Airways mobile toilets in Lagos rather than Soul City?'

'Exactly.' We both smile ruefully and then Pamela asks an odd question. 'Have you ever been into an old cathedral?'

'I have …' I reply, not sure where she's going with this. 'When I did A levels in London I sang in the choir in Westminster Abbey.'

'You did?' she says incredulously.

'Don't I look like a choir boy?'

'Maybe once!' she says with a smile. 'Anyway, did you know that cathedrals took multiple generations of artisans to build? The foundation builders knew they would never see their work complete, but they built anyway, content that what they were doing was for future generations.'

'I've never thought of that.'

'Well, I think your work is like those artisans, building for the future. Sometimes you'll be the tipping point that gets people to change; other times you may be simply part of their journey.'

'And we may never know,' I say.

'We may never know.'

For a minute or two we are both silent. Then, 'Remember I shared with you how the Jungle Doctor series of books influenced my life?' I ask. Pamela nods. 'Well if, in the 1950s, their author Dr Paul White was to have pondered their impact, he would have had to exclude me – I hadn't been born yet!'

'Precisely.' Pamela finishes her coffee, looks at her watch and stands up. 'Okay, we're meeting with the Gates people now. Shall we go?'

We walk back to the meeting room. Isaac is already there, and so is Sylvia Mathews, head of the Gates Foundation. I begin my pitch before Isaac does his. Unfortunately, I seem to lose Mathews as soon as I start talking. For a person who is more used to discussing new approaches to hygiene, I quickly realise the only thing of interest to her in a soap opera is the soap. I decide to change tack. I know the foundation has invested millions in vaccine development but very little in communication. In fact, I've often wondered what use a vaccine is if people either don't know about it or are afraid of it? So that's the question I ask Mathews. She seems a little surprised but she still doesn't get where I'm going.

'Of course, you need education campaigns to build demand, billboards, public service announcements, things like that,' she says.

I know that I am more likely to fall pregnant than to get funded by the Gates Foundation, so I throw caution to the wind. 'Don't you think that it's strange that while public health invests heavily in twenty-first century science, its approach to behaviour change has remained stuck in the Dark Ages?' I challenge her.

'So what are you suggesting?' she asks, trying to mask her irritation.

'As good scientists we should be looking for what type of communications are actually shaping our societies and then we should harness those.'

'And those are?'

'Well, they're certainly not billboards and fact sheets, which are better at littering highways than shifting behaviour.'

'And you think you know what *is* effective?'

'Story.'

'Story?' Her groomed eyebrows have gone up at least a centimetre.

'Yes, story: dramas, soap operas, documentaries, even prime-time news. In fact, any story that harnesses the emotions. Because it is emotions, not facts, that influence our behaviour.'

While Mathews seems unmoved, Pamela nods affirmingly and adds, 'Like all cultures through the ages.'

'That's right. Since we crawled out of our caves, we've used story to shape and transmit our norms and to make sense of our world. Instinctively we've sugar-coated life information so that the medicine goes down. But along the way somehow we seem to have lost the art.' I'm irritated and on a roll, so I just continue, whether the Gates woman is interested or not. 'If the evidence for the use of story is so overwhelming, why don't public health professionals get it? Is it because it's just too fluffy? Not exact enough? And yet there's a whole field of how to do this, and the evidence and the science to back it up.'

The silence in the room is as icy as the toboggan run but not nearly as exhilarating. How to win friends and influence people, I think.

Sylvia Mathews shrugs, before thanking me politely and turning to Isaac.

My pitch is over, as is my chance of funding.

Isaac goes full steam ahead with his toilets, widows and orphans.

'Oh, I love it!' Mathews exclaims, delighted to be on safer ground. 'And how much would it cost the foundation to sponsor some of your toilets?'

A thoughtful look comes over Isaac's broad face and then he says, '$300 each.'

'We'll take a thousand!'

Pamela and I share a smile at the Nigerian rate of inflation.

14.

BEYOND THE RIVER

Like a storm-tossed leaf, the narrow canoe bounces through the rapids of the Duzi River. Steve, his face a mask of agony and effort, shouts, 'One more!' as he stabs his blade into the water, urging them on. A double drumbeat sounds. In the front of the boat Duma momentarily disappears under a wall of water before he breaks through, water cascading off his muscular young body. The iconic sounds of Johnny Clegg's 'Impi' crescendo.

The image on the large screen pans out, a stretch of flat water that lies between Duma and Steve's boat and the finish. Only one canoe can stop their quest for a gold medal. The music trails away and is replaced by sounds of paddle splashes and ragged breathing.

All around me, in the darkened hall, people are clapping and shouting, willing the athletes on. The two boats draw level. Then, as if tethered to each other, the lead swaps by centimetres at a time. Through gritted teeth Duma shouts, 'Look the dog in the eye, Bra Steve!' Steve grimaces a smile. He knows the code: it's a call to stare down their devils with a final last effort. Then, with a unity of motion their boat breaks free. Now they are only a few paddle strokes to the line. A final sprint and they power under the finishing banner. Gold!

The audience erupts. People are standing up, shouting and cheering.

It's so strange. We know that this is just a film, but the story has blurred the lines between fiction and reality, pulling us into an emotional journey with these two men, divided by age and race, as they find a way to triumph. Our film *Beyond the River* has done what all well-told stories should do. It has captivated our imaginations and emotions. But will it spark the conversations we hope for? Will people be encouraged to get to know a little more about each other's stories? That is, after all, why Heartlines made it, as a building block for our 'What's Your Story?' campaign.

I leave the hall, blinking into the crisp morning light, transported from the Valley of a Thousand Hills to a wine farm in Franschhoek. In Harmonie is a retreat centre on the La Motte wine estate. Newly built, the centre is a triumph of new architecture meets old Cape Dutch. The buildings are nestled at the base of the valley and are encompassed by the ordered beauty of vineyards and lavender bushes before transitioning into fynbos-covered slopes that march up the surrounding grey-peaked mountains.

This time I am not on a personal crisis retreat or training to be a missionary in the field. Many years have passed since then.

Today I am meeting with 30 Christian leaders to contemplate how to help South Africans journey from racism and prejudice to reconciliation.

Rough place for a meeting, I think, as I take in the natural beauty that's all around me. If the going gets tough, at least the wine will be good.

There is a buzz of excited talk after the screening of the Heartlines' film. People are still high on the adrenalin of the finish.

I feel a hand on my shoulder and turn to see the smiling face of Moss Ntlha, the authoritative head of the Evangelical Alliance of South Africa. He takes off his thick glasses and wipes them on the hem of his shirt. His eyes are red rimmed. He clears his throat. 'I had heard it was good, but I wasn't expecting that … it was amazing.'

As I thank him, Olefile Masangane joins us. Ole is the head of Heartlines' church mobilisation. 'I told you, moruti, it's a film that makes you think, makes you realise how much we assume about each other.'

'True,' Moss agrees. 'What I really love about your approach is that you don't beat people over the head with a message. Rather you tell a story and let people do their own thinking. Very biblical!'

Ole and I glance at each other, relieved. We are often dismissed as not 'Christian' enough because we don't have any overt Christian messaging in our films.

'So, moruti, are you still happy that we spend the day getting this group to share their personal stories?' Ole asks.

Before he can answer, a tall, grey-haired man, reminiscent of an Old Testament prophet, joins us. This is Alexander 'Bushy' Venter, co-chair, with Moss, of this meeting and a pastor who, in the 80s, blazed a trail by setting up a mixed-race church in Soweto.

'I think we must,' Moss responds earnestly. 'Alexander, are you in agreement?'

'Absolutely!' Alexander says with conviction. 'As leaders we like producing declarations and pledges, but we don't have time for that now. I fear if we don't give ordinary people something tangible to do to cross the chasms of race and privilege, it may be too late for our country.'

The plan is to take a break for half an hour and then meet back at the hall. Before he leaves, Moss turns to me. 'As a matter of interest, Garth, how did Heartlines come up with this concept?'

I launch into our story of how, over the past few years, we had become concerned that the racial elephant in the room was growing and despite much well-meaning talk no one seemed to have a clue what to do. So we felt compelled to find a way for ordinary people to take action. We looked around the world and were surprised to find nothing, at least not at scale. Lots of small initiatives in places like Israel/Palestine, but that was it. I remember feeling really down. Perhaps there were no examples for a reason; perhaps it was just too hard.

Then, quite by chance, we found what we were looking for. In the process of our desire to build a more inclusive workplace, someone at the Heartlines office suggested that we take turns to tell our stories. It seemed like a fun thing to do, so with no great expectations, we went for it. As each story was told, the more surprised we became. I was particularly struck at how blindsided we all were as our assumptions about each other crashed and burned. I knew, for example, that Gosiame had a daughter but I didn't know that he was a single father, caring for his daughter because he didn't think her mother could. Or that Brian's family had been forcibly removed from the 'Coloured' area they were living in because they were white. It felt like for the first time people were seeing beyond stereotypes and, from a deeper understanding, trust was building. We had not set out to deal with race and reconciliation that day. It had surfaced naturally and in a non-threatening way.

We realised that was it. We would inspire and support millions (not just thousands) of people to get to know a little more about the stories of the people around them and make it a habit. Simple, wonderful, crazy!

'So that's how it came about, Moss,' I say, 'but we've gone much further. We've been developing "What's Your Story?" for the workplace and for schools and that's great, but unless we get the church to embrace and promote this in thousands of congregations we realise we will just be spitting into the wind.'

'So today is key,' Alexander asks, more statement than question.

'Today is key,' I reply.

'We back you guys, Garth, but don't be surprised if you meet some resistance in the storytelling session. People don't like being vulnerable,' Moss warns as he and Alexander go in search of coffee and Ole and I amble towards the meeting room.

'People's stories have power, right?' Ole looks at me quizzically. He's been around me enough to be unsure whether he wants to hear the rest. 'So once these guys experience it, this could really spread like we pray it will?' I nod.

'No pressure,' I say cheerfully. 'Just don't stuff it up.'

Ole smiles wanly. He will be responsible for facilitating 'What's Your Story?' with the group.

Our banter is interrupted as a woman walks over and greets us. Ole hugs her, then turns to me. 'Garth, this is Anneke from Piet Retief, remember I told you about her?'

Anneke is the archetypal Afrikaans farmer's wife. A dark-haired, big-boned woman with a significant presence. In fact, she is a farmer's wife, but that's where the stereotype ends. Anneke is a reconciler who has made it her life's work to be an active healer between black and white.

'I am so looking forward to today,' Anneke says. 'I've been praying for an opportunity to publicly repent for the sin of apartheid. When I heard that we had invited Mamphela Ramphele to join us, God placed on my heart the desire to ask her for forgiveness and permission to wash her feet.'

I cringe. My first thought is, flip, she can't be serious! But she is. I wonder why this makes me feel so uncomfortable. Is it because she will be dismissed as a white person looking for an easy way to assuage their guilt? Probably. But maybe that's my problem, not hers.

We walk into the hall. It's a bright, clean space. High, white ceilings are broken up by arching wooden trusses and curved windows that give a view onto the mountains.

We're late. The rest of the group are already seated.

I recognise a number of people, among them our Heartlines colleague Seth Naicker. Greying, in his mid-40s, Seth has a dress sense that sets a benchmark in Indie-African chic. There's old Bishop Bethlehem from Port Elizabeth, Reverend Angelo Scheepers, the long-standing head of the Baptist convention. Edwin Arrison and Peter Tarantal, both leaders from the Western Cape. The rest I don't know, but there is a mixture of age, race and gender.

The room feels a little tense, like when people are just about to write an exam. No one seems thrilled at the idea of sharing their stories. I worry about how is Ole going to handle this.

With skill is the answer. Taking the measure of his audience, Ole woos them by invoking the magic that has cracked ice since the dawn of time.

'I want to tell you a story,' he says.

The room is silent, the audience waiting.

'A man sat waiting for his flight to be called. To pass the time, he opened a packet of biscuits and ate one. To his surprise, the man next to him reached into the packet and smiled before taking one too. He couldn't believe it. Every time he took a biscuit, so did the man. Doing his best to conceal his irritation, the man reached for the last biscuit while keeping an eye on his neighbour. With a grin, the man gestured for him to take it. As if it was his to give! Trying hard to control his temper, the man stands up to leave. As he's reaching for his coat, he sees a packet of unopened biscuits on his seat. He's beyond embarrassed! All this time he had been eating his neighbour's biscuits! And to make matters worse the guy had been so nice about it!'

There is a ripple of uncomfortable laughter.

'I often judge people without knowing their full story,' Ole says, 'and then I find myself embarrassed by my preconceptions. Sound familiar?'

Aware that the mood has shifted, Ole then says quietly, 'Okay, I want you to put aside your anxiety and give story-sharing a go. If, after trying it, you feel it's not for you, we'll ditch it and move onto something else. But first, I'm going to tell you my story. As I do, I want you to really listen because when you listen you are communicating to me without words; you're telling me that I'm important to you. It's like the Zulu greeting "Sawubona": I see you.'

There is silent consent.

'I was born in a little village called Lehurutse in the former Bophuthatswana. My mother worked as a domestic worker and raised us by herself ...'

Although I've heard his story before, as Ole begins, taking us into the dusty streets of his childhood, each time I gain a deeper level of understanding and respect for who he is, for what he has overcome to become the man, father and husband that he is today. Although we come from different worlds, there is so much that we share as son, husband and father.

As the day progresses the sense of greater understanding among people is tangible. People who've known each other for years are astonished at how little they actually know about each other. There are plenty of stories of triumph and of pain. What is clear is that your race or gender exclude you from neither. There is a rawness that is sometimes uncomfortable but feels so real; it is unlike the interactions many of us are so used to having, where we skirt along the fringes of each other's lives.

However, there are still pockets of chill, supressed anger, heightened by what some may be perceiving – that the act of sharing stories is a cop-out, an easy way to assuage guilt. Perhaps they feel their pain requires something more radical than storytelling. I doubt, outside of forgiveness, that they will find the balm they seek.

The day is also interspersed with humour as people recount some of the ridiculous stuff that makes up life. There is laughter when I recount how, all the way through medical school, I fainted at the sight of blood and how it was so bad that when I was about to deliver my first baby, I passed out. Only a timely leap from my student partner saved the baby from falling.

When I share my journey with anxiety and depression and my naming what I suffer from SHS (Stuffed Head Syndrome) there is amusement, as I intend there to be, but there is also appreciation for my vulnerability, which in turn enables others to be freer in sharing their own struggles. I realise that no matter how often I share my story, I seem to gain a deeper insight into myself while giving a gift to others. If they find inspiration in my story and the courage to share their own, I will feel like I have achieved something good

However, I often feel vulnerable in sharing my story with people I hardly know. I am pretty secure in who I am, but there is always the nagging thought, what will people think of me when they know the truth? Many people feel like this, especially as they transition from a time of deep vulnerability back into the mundanities of life. One minute someone is sharing about being abused, next you are asking her to pass the biscuits. Knowing this, Ole alerts us to how we may feel and encourages us to have the courage to be comfortable with being uncomfortable, the personal risk being far less than the potential reward.

When Anneke tells her story, I begin to understand what has led her to so passionately promote forgiveness and reconciliation. She shares how she had to forgive her husband and reconcile with him when she found out there was a third person in her marriage. She describes how she felt that God had used her pain to open her eyes to the pain and suffering of many black people caused by 'her people' and her resultant conviction to make amends.

As the afternoon draws to a close, Mamphela stands up and begins to tell her story. Her slight build belies the steel that enabled her to take on and triumph over both politicians and police. With grace and style she takes us on the journey of her life. It feels like we are reliving history. We move with her from her birth in the Bochum district of Limpopo to her medical studies and student activism in the apartheid 70s. She describes her relationship with and then loss of Steve Biko. And so she continues with her remarkable story.

'Did you ever give up hope?' Seth asks.

'Never,' she replies. 'I knew we would either be free or die. I hoped for the one and didn't fear the other.' She gives us a dry smile.

'And are you bitter at the people who did this to you?' Seth asks.

'Sad, yes, bitter, no. I'm grateful for a faith that shows the wisdom of forgiveness.'

Anneke is sitting opposite me. Next to her are two Afrikaans women, Corne and Lynette. They hold hands tightly, struggling to contain their emotions. Ole walks over to Anneke. 'Perhaps now is the time to ask her?' he says gently. She hesitates, looks at him and then slowly stands and walks over to Mamphela.

Time is suspended. All eyes are fixed on them. Anneke bends down and takes Mamphela's small hands in hers. In a barely audible voice she says, 'Mamphela, would you forgive me and my people for what we have done to you and yours?' Her voice breaks as she continues, 'And would you allow me to wash your feet as an act of repentance?' Mamphela pauses in thought before, eyes glistening, she gives a nod of assent.

'Tonight, after dinner then?' Ole says, breaking a moment that feels both sacred and uncomfortable.

Through the day, I have felt like a sports coach, totally invested in the game but powerless to affect the outcome. Hyped when I see people 'get it' and bummed when I see that others don't. I still don't know what the final score will be.

Ole is sensitive to the rhythm of the day, which has produced both converts and sceptics. He knows that more time will not change that. So with the room turning golden as the sun dips behind the mountains, he thanks us. 'Enjoy your dinner, but since we are at a wine farm I ask the Baptists to watch over our Anglican and Catholic brothers and sisters, lest they be tempted by the spirit.' He knows his audience and his in-house Christian humour elicits smiles, allowing people to transition out of the intensity of the day.

Ole, Seth and I cluster together as people walk out into the dusk in companionable groups.

'So?' Ole says, looking at me.

'So what?' I respond, deadpan.

'Don't mess with me, Garth!'

I love it when Ole is exasperated, but this time I decide to let him off the hook. 'I thought you were masterful the way you handled them,' I say. 'Not easy. Still not sure whether we will get their full backing, but that is between them and God.'

'Ja, broer – a master class!' Seth confirms, gripping Ole's shoulder, before turning to me. 'Garth, you're an Anglican, right?'

'Sometimes,' I respond.

'We'll be watching you!' he says with a grin.

As we turn to leave, Moss, Peter, Alexander and Edwin walk up to us, looking serious. I feel like I am waiting for my parent to open my school report. What will they say?

'We have been chatting,' Moss begins in a measured voice, 'and felt that we should give you some feedback.' Like a good preacher, Moss uses pause to great effect and he stops talking. Sensing my anxiety, he laughs. 'Don't worry, it was amazing! Look, we have to discuss it more broadly but you've convinced us that we need to get behind "What's Your Story?" It's simple, practical and transformative.'

We are elated!

'Come – dinner waits,' Moss says as they turn to go.

Tonight I'm an Anglican.

15.

HEARTLINES

The name we had originally decided on for the new organisation was Heartlands and I loved it – except that when I did a web search I discovered it was taken. It was the name of an upmarket … shall we say, adult store – probably more profitable than we would ever be!

So Heartlines, representing the values that make us human and connect our hearts, we became. The values we identified, and by which we still live, are:

Compassion
Self-control
Forgiveness
Grace
Perseverance
Honesty
Acceptance
Responsibility

'Remember these values are only for the general public,' I tell my colleagues, often. 'In these offices they're just for decoration.' Which always gets an eye-roll. They've become adept at ignoring me. Unsurprising, really. It's hard to treat a CEO who keeps a loaded master-blaster water-pistol at his desk seriously.

We have come a long way since that first meeting with World Vision and the road was not without its potholes. There was many a setback we found ourselves having to contend with and find creative ways around.

Our first Heartlines campaign, 'Eight weeks, Eight Values, One National Conversation', hit South Africa's screens in 2006. It comprised a set of eight TV films, each dealing with a different value, and each film was shown on all three SABC channels simultaneously, something that had never been done before. We reached over 12 million people.

In a similar way to our Soul City vision having the broadest reach possible on multiple platforms and a variety of media, the films were preparing the ground for the seed. As I had described it to my tutor Claire that day after my 'hillock experience', the films prepare the field. Our committed and creative team developed and produced complementary written resources for thousands of churches, schools and prisons, underpinning the values as demonstrated in visual form in the films.

It was a roller-coaster time, full of adrenalin highs and confounding troughs. You could say the challenge of translating a fluffy concept, of wanting to inspire people to live their better selves into a concrete project, was 'interesting' . The further challenges of being in production with eight films simultaneously, getting a then elderly Nelson Mandela to introduce them, and getting them broadcast on all SABC channels at the same time confounds even me, as I think back on it now.

'You want to do what?' and 'It's never been done before' had apparently not deterred me. Years ago, I'd heard something similar …

In addition to the print material, we set up discussions on the films with nine different language radio stations, produced weekly print opinion pieces, a music CD, and an illustrated children's storybook in eleven languages. Then came the task of engaging with the 'organised' church – an oxymoron – to prepare them for the eight-week period. Initially, this took the form of mailing out a discussion guide blindly to 60 000 congregations so that they could engage with the films. Never has the expression 'spray and pray' been so apt!

This was work for 30 people but in the beginning there were only four harried souls. Harried both by the extent of what we'd taken on and by me rushing into the offices, creating havoc and then escaping back to my full-time job at Soul City. There were so many times I wanted to chuck the whole thing in, only to pull back at the last moment because I did not want to let down the extraordinary people who had given so much.

All these years later, people still talk about the impact the series had on them. The films and resources are still used today in schools, churches and prisons throughout South Africa.

But at the time, like the proverbial dog that has caught the bus, after this initial campaign I was at a loss as to what to do next. I had always relied on the next cat's eye in the road appearing at the right time, confident that even if the destination was vague, there was a destination and that I could rely on God to get me there.

This time, however, what our next move would be remained elusive. I'd always taken comfort in having a vision, a story to pursue, even if it was a crazy idea. Without one, I was stuck in the swirling mist; waiting for it to lift was futile. I was at a loss. It was a depressing period. Even thinking about it now is horrible. I scrambled around for a compelling vision, but the more I sought one, the mistier the future seemed to become.

Eventually, it came to me that our next campaign should be to promote civic values. We called this campaign 'Values in Action', an initiative to help people live their values though community action. We headlined it with a TV miniseries, Hopeville, which would receive much acclaim. It would be nominated for an international Emmy and go on to win the prestigious Rose d'Or. Hopeville was supported by resources for churches and schools, including a children's book, like those we had produced for our initial eight films.

Along with my vision for a campaign to promote civic values came the recognition that an additional platform, a digital one, was a necessity. This would be the game changer. Heartlines would embrace the twenty-first century and build a digital platform to connect people to the needs of organisations already doing good work. It was to do so much more. It would rival Facebook for functionality.

We called the platform 'forgood'.

The relief I felt in having a way forward was indescribable, but what followed was a nightmare. The films and the resources were successful but the foray into the digital space was a humbling of my arrogance. I'd thought that if I could dream it, I could do it. Raise money. Find some software developers. Get them to build the platform – how hard could it be? Very, was the answer. We proceeded to pour our collective energies into its creation. It cost a fortune, took ages and … it didn't work.

The worst was the impact on my colleagues. They'd trustingly believed my vision and its failure cast a pall over us all. My depression almost overwhelmed me. I dreamed of a new job, one where the outcomes were more tangible, but I knew I couldn't leave. I believed even when I didn't that there was a reason for Heartlines.

I'm reminded how affirming it can be to retrace one's story. What felt disastrous then has ultimately been a success. Forgood is now the largest volunteering platform in the country, a profitable company majority-owned by Heartlines. It was a game changer, yes. But the lessons learned in building it were tough ones.

AT MEDICAL SCHOOL we did an experiment to see whether with a blindfold and peg on our noses we could tell the difference between Coke, Fanta and Sprite. To my surprise, it was impossible, such is the importance of these senses to taste.

But coffee! That's different. Deprive me of all my senses and I would still recognise coffee, because of the way it makes me feel. Awake. I'm not an addict, I don't think, but in the morning my neurons seem barely to stutter along until they are prodded into action by the miraculous brown bean.

Kick-starting my neurons is a pleasurable ritual. Each morning I walk into the office and prepare a large mug of Bean There Ethiopian coffee and a slice of toast that creaks under the weight of peanut butter. Then I retreat to a quiet place to contemplate life and the universe.

Today that quiet place is our boardroom to wait for the welcome sounds of my colleagues, who will be making their way here shortly.

The boardroom is not large, but it's big enough for 30 of us to sit around the table. Three burnt-orange walls are offset by a purple carpet, a tribute to our Heartlines colours. The third wall is made up mostly of a window that looks out onto busy Jan Smuts Avenue. On a shelf below the window is a collection of statues, the prestigious awards we have received for our films. On one of the walls are eight square wood cuts, each with a word carved into it – our Heartlines values.

Our gathering together here once a week has become a central feature of Heartlines' culture. Each week a person tells their story – sometimes in great depth, sometimes superficially, but never failing to give us greater insight into one another. It began as an experiment some years back as a way to build understanding between our team and is now the highlight of our week. It also became the basis for our national 'What's Your Story?' campaign to build understanding among ordinary South Africans.

Today it will be Gosiame's turn.

I take a seat in one corner while the boardroom is still empty and settle in with my toast and coffee, allowing my mind to drift back to when Heartlines began. I can scarcely believe it, but it was 14 years ago, and 24 years since I first had the idea. Just remembering it all makes me tired. I look at the wood cuts and contemplate their meaning as I sip my coffee, savouring the aroma. As I feel my neurons yawning and stretching, grateful for their caffeine kick, gratitude floods through me. While the intervening years have had their crises, I've never again felt like we've lost our way. There's been more joy than desperation and it seems that the cats' eyes are shining brighter now, pointing us towards an exciting and more impactful future.

In later years when the COVID-19 pandemic turns all our worlds upside down, it will feel like a switch has been flipped and the cats' eyes snuffed out. We will battle to navigate Heartlines into the unknown, but will feel reassured by remembering the road we have travelled. We will have faith that the next cat's eye will emerge.

I'm shaken out of my reverie by the sound of the boardroom door opening, heralding the arrival of the variety of people who make up the Heartlines staff. We are every shade and gender. Some might be what you'd call vertically challenged, while others are built for comfort and not for speed. Some are at the end of their careers and others just starting out. Some have been dealt a rough hand in life and there are others whose lives have been less challenging. But all are committed to what we do. They are why I am still here.

Zamabongo, the super-talented, fun and passionate head of our values and money campaign, peers at me through her dreads. 'Good morning, Garthy,' she says. She always calls me that, I'm not sure why. Thabisa, our regal head of human resources, is the next to walk in.

As the boardroom fills up, the noise level rises. When everyone is seated, Tina, our receptionist, shushes us. We all love Tina. Despite what are sometimes difficult circumstances, she always seems to radiate joy and we pay attention when she calls us to order. 'Today,' she reminds us, 'Gosiame is going to share his story. Even though some of you may have heard the story before, listen well.'

A familiar hush, elicited by the magical anticipation of a story, settles over the room.

Gosiame is a lanky man in his late 30s. He sits down at the end of the table. Ayanda gamely attempts to wire him up to be recorded, while he vigorously stirs his coffee. As Tina has said, some of us have heard the story of how he became a chicken murderer a few times but we don't mind hearing it again.

Gosiame is a natural storyteller and he has a flair for drama and he always introduces a few new twists and turns. The responses when he is finished from those who are hearing his story for the first time are often the same, as are his explanations: 'Eish, man! No you didn't!' ('We had to, baba, we had no choice, how else were we going to get meat?') A collective intake of breath accompanied by nervous giggles. Newcomers who have had a sheltered upbringing nearly always ask: 'But why the nail up the chicken's bum?' which elicits a broad smile from the storyteller. ('Because then you can't see how the chicken died. My uncle would think that the chicken had been sick and so would then tell my brother and I to throw it away. "Sure, baba," we would say and then we would run into the bush and braai it.')

Gosiame's narrative gifting transports us to the world of his youth.

'This was not the life we knew,' he says without bitterness. 'In ekasi we had shoes, we had food. I would say to my uncle, "I want such and such", and he would get it. When he died everything changed for my brother and I. Our mother couldn't keep us, so she sent us to relatives outside of Rustenburg. Yoh, that was a shock. We became like their slaves. Us city boys, my younger brother and I, suddenly in the bundus looking after chickens and cattle.'

The only movement and sound in the room is Gosiame still violently stirring his coffee.

'Eish, the winters were the worst,' he continues. 'We had no shoes. We would wait for a cow to do its business and then quickly put our feet into the steaming pile. Eish, that was good.'

Ayanda can't help herself. She reaches across and grabs the spoon from Gosiame's hand. He looks at her, startled. 'I'm trying to record this and you're making noise with the spoon!' she hisses.

Suitably chastised, Gosiame continues with his tale. It is a hard story. The rural uncle dies and he returns to the city. His mother tries to care for her children, but without work, she resorts to the option chosen by many poor and desperate woman – men. Gosiame tells his story with humour but his pain is evident. 'She didn't have to travel far from home,' he says with a sad smile. 'All the men were from the neighbourhood. Four of us, each with a different father. She died when I was still very young. The other children went to their fathers, but not me. My father did not want me.' Around the room tears are welling. 'I thought I'm a nobody, worth nothing. I had no hopes so I had no fears. I went wild. This was the 80s and the army was in the townships, we comrades, 'Sayinyova,' were burning tyres and hijacking trucks. Yoh, the best were the beer trucks – we would be drunk all weekend! We would throw stones at the white soldiers and they would shoot at us. I learned to hate white people.' He looks around the room, his gaze coming to rest on Derek. 'But not anymore.'

Tall and grey haired, Derek is an accountant in his mid-60s. He took early retirement from his senior executive job at Nedbank, where he had a massive office, a massive desk, a knee-high carpet, and hot and cold running assistants. Thankfully, he agreed to join Heartlines and took up a tiny workspace in the passage.

Derek and Gosiame developed a unique bond when they understood that their stories intersected. While Gosiame was throwing stones at white soldiers, Derek realised that he might well have been one of those soldiers. In a wonderful way, this shared history has been healing for them both.

'I was heading one way, baba,' admits Gosiame. 'If the Salvation Army had not offered me a place, I think I would be dead by now. I met a man there who, for the first time in my life, was interested in me not for what I could do for him but for who I was. I am not sure what it was he saw in me but that man became the father I never had. "Gosiame," he would say, "I believe in you." Just to know that this man thought I was good enough, saved me.'

Gosiame's is an extraordinary story. It is hard to equate the man he is today with the wild, fatherless youth he describes.

'Why didn't your dad want you?' Pam asks.

That it is Pam asking the question is not surprising. Pamela Kgare, open faced with a beautiful smile, is the colleague heading up the development of our next campaign, which is promoting the active, positive presence of men in the lives of children. We're in the discovery phase of the project where we are getting stories and asking questions. Why is it that over 60 per cent of the children in South Africa are growing up without fathers? Only after we understand the answers better can we hope to have an impact.

While that is the main motivation for Pam's question, I know it's also personal. She was rejected by her father, too, and wants to know why.

'I don't know,' Gosiame says. We can see this is hard for him. 'I phoned him and he pretended not to know who I was. I didn't want money or anything, I just wanted to meet him.' Even as an adult, the wound of his father's rejection is evident.

Gosiame's story echoes the hundreds of stories we have heard. The majority of both men and women believe that a man's primary role is to provide money. If he can't, then the woman doesn't see a role for him. 'I don't want another child to care for' is a common refrain we have heard from these women. And because the man doesn't see a role for himself, he moves on.

As Gosiame has experienced his life turning around, he dedicates it to being present in the lives of people like him who may never have known affirmation. He is also a single dad, determined to be the father that he never had to his daughter.

'Yoh, baba, I'm out of time,' Gosiame says, glancing at his watch. There is a collective groan. Gosiame's story has been truly stranger than fiction. We're barely out of his childhood and we all want to hear more. But our desks and our telephones are calling and we reluctantly accept that we can't sit and listen to his story all day. Tina thanks Gosiame and prays for him. She expresses the gratitude that we all feel. His shared story has been an act of generosity, placing some of our struggles into perspective and giving hope to others.

As my colleagues entered into the room so they process out, a loud gaggle of disparate humanity.

Alone with my thoughts, I sit for a bit longer, enjoying the warm morning sunshine, reflecting on Gosiame's story and how often people's stories are mostly about their childhood. I suppose it's no surprise, given that these are our formative years. However, what does surprise me is how many people have had either physically or emotionally absent fathers and how difficult that has been for them. They often struggle to articulate why they have found this is so painful. My sense is that as children we all, men and women, have the innate need to be affirmed by a loving man. Seemingly, the need for a father's blessing is hard-wired into our DNA.

Could it be that there are some formative pieces of our journey from child to adult, which only the presence of an affirming loving man can put in place? The absence of those pieces seems to have a profound impact on some people. Many spend their lives searching for them, often in the wrong places.

I shiver slightly at the outrage that is bound to be the reaction to these sentiments. What about the millions of women successfully raising children on their own, no man in sight? I am battling with the challenge we face. How do we balance the overwhelming evidence that children need to have the influence of good men in their lives, without undermining the extraordinary work of single mothers? Like smoking is a risk factor for cancer, this, too, is a risk for children. It increases their risk of being victims or perpetrators of violence, abusing substances, teenage pregnancy, mental illness and poor academic performance. But it's a risk, not a sentence, as millions of successful adults will attest.

It's a challenge I know we will and must face. I pray for the wisdom to do so. Backing away from this is not an option. I think about how struck I was by an article that quoted leading researchers as saying that absent fathers is one of the biggest challenges facing the world, outranking even poverty.

I pause my thoughts to wonder why I feel more passionately about this particular issue than another? I have a burning desire to use what I've learned over the last 27 years to ensure that more men are actively, positively involved in the lives of children. Perhaps it's because everything else I've been involved in, like HIV/AIDS and gender-based violence, are not things I have experienced personally. This issue I can explore from a personal perspective, however.

I think about my relationship with my dad. I can't believe it's been ten years since he died. I know that when I started to make sense of my story, I'd been angry at him for not challenging my mother's pathological attachment to me. If he had, things would have been different, I felt. I was sad that for so many years I'd been desperate to feel that I was good enough, that my father was proud of me, but it was only towards the end of his life that I felt I'd received his blessing.

The years have passed now and I have come to feel a profound gratitude to my father. He never had the example of a present father. In fact, the only thing his father seemed to excel at was getting married. My grandfather was married five times. It seems that he used his position as Johannesburg's leading divorce lawyer to scout out his next wife. Did Dad ever have his father's blessing? I doubt it, and yet my father did the best he could. I never wanted for anything materially and he ensured that I had an excellent education. But his greatest gifts to me were his examples of generosity, of respect for all people and fear for none, and his desire for social justice.

My chief regret as I sit here this morning alone in the empty boardroom is that I never made time to ask my father for his story. Yes, I got fragments, but not the sort of dedicated time I'd spent getting my mother's story, and I know how profoundly that changed my understanding of her.

I wonder how my own children will reflect on their father. Am I present enough? Am I supportive and affirming enough? Eish! I am sure like my parents before me I will mess up. Hopefully, as they learn my story, they will understand me better and that will make all the difference.

'We are meeting now and you are in my chair.' Zamabongo strides purposefully into the boardroom in one of her 20 pairs of All Stars and stands over me. 'Do you remember the ninth Heartlines value?' she asks.

I'm flummoxed.

'It is more blessed to go than to remain!'

There is no reply to that so I unfold myself and take my leave.

IN OTHERS' WORDS ...

Brent Lindeque discovered through the power of social media how you can take something socially fun but more destructive than useful and turn it on its head. His moment of insight came when he was challenged during an early viral craze around 2014 called Neknomination. Essentially, it was a drinking game. It originated in New Zealand but soon swept the world like a wildfire out of control. You would drink a lot of alcohol while doing something silly somewhere in the world and then 'nominate' a friend to go one better. 'The idea was to drink as much as you possibly could,' said Brent. 'There were millions of people uploading these videos.' At the time, 'there were a couple of things going through my head. One was that as South Africans we face other problems that first world countries do not have. The second was why aren't we using social media to be more responsible? Our biggest problems are unemployment, poverty and crime. They all sit in one bubble. When I was Neknominated, instead of drinking and challenging people to do the same, I decided to film myself doing random acts of kindness to homeless people instead.

'I put my first video on YouTube and by that evening it had 10 000 views and the next morning 100 000. All of a sudden, CNN wanted to interview me, then Australia Morning Live and, locally, 702 and eNCA. There was an interest and the interest was not me. The story was about how an average South African changed the social media game and how suddenly all over the world there were these people who were just doing random acts of kindness. They were sharing goodness and doing beautiful things. Even in the first world. They were looking after the broken people in society and it was humbling to watch.'

Out of a long and successful career in marketing, advertising, brand building and consulting, Ivan Moroke knows better than most the power of persuasion. One of his passions is transformation. Being so close to advertising, Ivan was well aware that the industry had huge issues with transformation. After democracy in 1994 and after our new Constitution came into effect in 1997, 'there were new laws, new charters that were done that the advertising agencies were supposed to live by' – but he believed that the key lay in collaboration. Wouldn't it be great, he thought, if besides what they have *got* to do, they can do it willingly? He saw the inherent value in Heartlines' 'What's Your Story?' programme as a means of getting people to understand one another. Apart from transformation being a goal in the industry, for companies who wanted to advertise and sell their products there was a strong commercial imperative. 'Understanding transformation is a critical business success factor because you have to understand people. If you do not have people who might understand the people you are trying to talk to, it does not make sense.'

Ivan took the 'What's Your Story?' programme and ran with it. Through sharing their personal stories in a professionally facilitated environment, in small workshops as well as larger groups, the effects were palpable. He found some of the responses from black people hearing their colleagues' stories for the first time especially interesting.

'After the stories were told, they would say, "I would not have known." There were different groups and workshops. Some would say, "In this group, I actually find that I have got more in common with someone who, because of their race, I never would have thought I had." They might actually have less in common with another black person in the group. That was a fundamental thing to say. In the end it proves what we have always known – that humans are similar. Leaving aside the personality front and maybe history or background, humans want the same things. It is as simple as that at the end of the stories. They may have what they call their values, like the best for their family, aspirations and all that stuff. At the end, it is what it comes down to. It is not surprising that there were surprises, if you know what I mean. It is not surprising that people were surprised that I am so similar to you in terms of how I view life.'

In my interview with Jonathan Robinson, we talked about leadership and the effect of using 'What's Your Story?' with staff and colleagues. 'As a company we have really tried to get to know each other's story. We have also opened up a comfortable environment for people to say how they feel, which is sometimes uncomfortable as a result. So I think we broke the seal on some racial issues. As a result people are free and I think we have a good and sometimes hard environment. Sometimes people will say it how they see it and that is hard.

'When I sat down and listened to the first stories in the group I was participating in, one staff member's story stuck significantly with me. He is perpetually late, he is always getting stabbed by his girlfriend and he makes many bad choices. In any other environment, he would have been fired for sure. He has been so unreliable at times that I should have fired him. Getting to know his story made all the difference in how I understand him. I still have to be hard and tell him what is not acceptable but it gave me awareness and, I guess, increased grace towards him, once I understood. He had no parents or siblings and was brought up unwanted on his aunt's property. His family would eat and not offer him food. He had to go scrounge for himself in the street and hustle so that he could eat when he was in a family structure that should have been providing food for him. I had new respect for his situation. Now that he is earning good money, he supports that family.'

Buhle Dlamini is another person who had it tough growing up. And, like many others, he has experienced stereotyping and racial profiling first-hand. He was raised by his grandparents in rural Hlabisa, then went to school in Durban, where he lived with his father in a back room until matric. When his father became unemployed, through his church, the Salvation Army (where he was one of the only black congregants), he moved into the home of a white Scots couple, who showed him only love and acceptance.

'I went from a rural background, living only with black people and then going into a mixed space and finding myself in 1995, living with this white family. When you think about the Rugby World Cup, I am watching it with the Petherbridges ... And all those other changes that were taking place in South Africa. My own experiences with racism even in my church come from that era but it is also confusing because you are facing racism from some people and you receive extraordinary love and acceptance from others. I guess that is a South African story in a big way. When I walk into any room, in the first five seconds people make a decision about who I am and my connections. In South Africa, if you are in the professional spaces and you are a young black person there are all kinds of assumptions. They think that maybe you went to a private school, come from a rich family or you are connected politically. When I tell my story, it shuts down all those stereotypes and creates a possibility for people to have an open blank space, which would allow them to connect with me.'

As an adult with his own family, Buhle continued to confound stereotypical thinking and assumptions. In doing his professional presentations to a variety of audiences, both in South Africa and abroad, and being always sensitive to tone and timing, he integrates his personal story. 'The way that I look at presenting and speaking is that it is more about the transition the audience goes through. From the beginning of the presentation to the end. The beginning of the presentation starts with an introduction of who I am. Typically I would say, "Hi, my name is Buhle Dlamini, as you have heard. I am married, with four kids." From there I speak about being married to a Canadian, having four children and the first one being in her 20s and I am 39. There is that confusion of doing the math and then I talk about how she was adopted; then I speak about my brother, and then our first biological child.

'We have a Congolese daughter with very distinct central Africa features, and then I look very much like Nhlanhla – my younger brother who we adopted – and then my wife Stacey is a blonde Canadian and our younger children are of mixed race.'

If anyone understands the power of story to effect change and challenge assumptions it is Buhle.

'That is where the real power of story comes,' he told me when we talked about this. 'Because not only does it get in touch with our emotions, but it also gets us in touch with our aspirations and what we actually want to do now that we know.' In his experience when he speaks on international platforms or performs his dramatic renditions bringing to life those in the past who have fought for justice and freedom, afterwards the conversation will often turn to race – although, as he explained, it could as easily be about poverty. The stereotyping is the point. 'If you have always thought that poor people are lazy and so on, and then you hear the story and it shuts your stereotype. You see the person behind the story, you understand their journey and all of a sudden your logic is overpowered by empathy. That moves you from thinking that poor people are lazy and not wanting to interact with them to becoming an activist for the poor. That is what is powerful about story. That it does not just change how we think about things. It changes what we do going forward.'

He told me about an experience he had with an audience in Germany some years ago. 'We saw that getting people to see beyond what they have been told, what they believe they know and what they believe is the truth about the other, and come to their own experience of the story about the other, where it is unfiltered – they see the human in the other person and see themselves in the other. When people are able to see the joys, pain, the raw human experience of the other, beyond the stereotypes, there is an Aha! moment that we are actually not different. Sometimes it is connecting with the heart; someone feels something for the other. It is not just sympathy but connection.' In the German audience that night there were a group of skinheads who, Buhle could tell, had come along with the intention of disrupting the show, of disrespecting the performers. Instead, the group were disarmed through the process that followed.

'We had a long discussion about why they hated foreigners they had never met. At the end of those conversations and having made those connections, they were the ones escorting us out of town,' Buhle laughed. 'That for me is a vivid experience of going from dislike and pure hate to a moment of connecting and engaging to now I am going to be a part of a different story going forward.'

Lillian Dube and David Dennis, through their many years as actors on Soul City, can both testify to how inhabiting a character and driving a story-line carries into a community and influences thousands, millions, of those who get pulled into drama and story. This resonates with the conversation I had with Sue Goldstein and Shereen Usdin all those years back and the term 'parasocial interaction', where people identify so strongly with characters that they can't distinguish between the drama on screen and real life. For Lillian, in becoming Sister Bettina, she remains Sister Bettina for many to this day.

'I was real,' she said. 'I was no longer Lillian Dube. Even to this day. That boy who composed the song "Sister Bettina" got it from there. I went to Sun City in 2018 and when the DJ saw me, he played the song.' Another time, when Lillian was in a bank, 'this gentleman came up to me – there was a time when we did a series on domestic violence ... and Patrick Shai played it so well – and this gentleman said to me, "Mama, thank you so much. I have stopped beating my wife because I saw myself in that." We addressed those issues back then and they are still happening today. What was painful for me was that Matlakala, who played Patrick's wife, was going through stuff. Playing that role was traumatising for her because she said that that was her mother's life. Even Patrick Shai went through that, which is why whenever he talks about it he gets emotional.

'There was an episode where I stopped Aubrey from smoking and people believed that and some even stopped. Even how the clinics are so far and people need to travel long distances to get or use the services, Soul City addressed those issues. Something as simple as not putting a primus stove on the table with a tablecloth when you have toddlers, not putting paraffin in cold drink bottles – we taught those things.'

David Dennis and Lillian are perhaps what you might call the stalwarts of that era. David reminisced about his role as Sol, and 'a storyline around a man that was living a reality of having to deal with what it was to be HIV-positive. First, by being ostracised in its broader sense but specifically losing his job, lover, wife and girlfriend. He was ostracised by family and then the immediate community on this basis of misunderstanding or non-understanding of what it actually meant to be HIV-positive.'

It was a brave role to take on at a time in South Africa where the stigma around AIDS and being HIV-positive was very real. 'The thing of going down the street and people saying "That is that guy who has AIDS," and suddenly it was like this is the only person who has AIDS in the country,' David said. 'It was a very interesting journey for me. On the one hand, that sometimes made it confusing, but, on the other, it made me talk to people and people could come and talk to me. People would come to me and say, "I have a friend. Can I ask you some questions?" People would come to my house and knock on the gate. Only over a decade or so, people started to differentiate between a character and the actor who portrayed the character. I had to occupy the space and be that person. Talk to people, to the point where I requested to go on a course personally – an HIV-counselling course.'

In a storyline in the third series of Soul City, which was when David joined the cast, Sol, angry and scared at just having been diagnosed as HIV-positive, took drastic action. 'His revenge was to take it out on the clinic where he was diagnosed.' What resulted was a dramatic hostage drama (which is still talked about, more than 20 years later), but it was the follow through that David highlights as critical. After the hostage drama ended, Sol's 'punishment' was to perform community service and he became an HIV counsellor. 'So that very important intervention was introduced,' said David. 'A very clever device was introduced so that people now, because we were accessing stories on the national broadcaster in our own language, now we were learning through this process. That intervention was important. I cannot stress that enough.'

David remembered doing a talk on domestic violence, when that was another storyline that was emerging. 'It was around December – the fourteen days of activism against abuse. I will never forget the courage of a woman who came up to me and spoke about her relationship with her husband. How it was affecting her, the family and children, his infidelities. Asking me what she should do and how she should go about protecting herself.' David Dennis the actor was a total stranger to this woman, but Sol, the character he played, was not. 'It was a task I had to accept,' David said.

'I think story becomes transformative in the way the messaging unfolds. Change is happening as we are listening. It is real. You feel it, you taste it, and it is there. People have said to me, "We will never forget you. You educated us. You taught us things we never knew." These are people who are now in their 50s or 60s.'

It is humbling when I hear these affirming stories about Soul City. I think back to the germ of an idea that grew into a crazy vision, which somehow became a reality. All of it is about story, the gift of story, how it is received and packaged in any manner of formats, how stories connect people and transform lives.

For David Dennis, the importance of using story to be transformative is critical. It is his mantra, he told me. 'That you are not just a storyteller for the sake of storytelling. It is your responsibility to transform our society. To change thinking and to challenge set ways of doing business. What is the point of telling a story unless if it is going to bring some change? Even if it is just one person. Just in general and in terms of my own experience of being an actor, the challenge I gave myself was a minimum of one. Affect at least one person. You do not abuse the trust and the responsibility you have been given as an artist. To get on to that stage and not just get bums on seats but to get them feeling something when they leave that place.'

Whether you are in the business of marketing a product or trying to make positive changes in a marginal community, it might seem basic that listening to the customer or the community is fundamental, but this is certainly not always the case.

Alison Harris uses the term 'human-centred design thinking'. 'So many solutions are formed from offices and from sitting behind a desk or just reading a story and not finding out more. So you start with empathising. You start with actually hearing someone's story before you even come up with any solutions. You are literally just listening to someone sharing. From there, you start defining what the problem or opportunity is. Then you start moving into the idea phase. From there you build a prototype – whether it is a system or product – and from there, you implement and test. It is circular.'

This resonated strongly with me and I mentioned Heartlines' current big project, about promoting men's active presence in the lives of children and the importance of the research process. We spend an entire year just listening. Only then do we begin to create a programme or intervention, which we will test with the people we are trying to reach before we implement it.

Jonathan Robinson uses the stories of the coffee growers that Bean There Coffee Company buys from as the central pillar of his marketing strategy. I asked him to define the term 'direct fair trade' for me. 'It's a process of trading fairly and directly with farmers,' he explained. 'So for us it means having a direct relationship with small-scale farmers in Ethiopia, Kenya, Rwanda, Burundi, Tanzania and the DRC. It is establishing long-term relationships. A big part of Bean There's story is connecting with communities, year in, year out. To be there for them in ups and downs and, hopefully, as a result they are there for us too and the relationship works both ways. We like people to get to know a country through its coffee. One of the reasons why we visit the farmers is so that we can come back and tell stories. People connect far more with the person in the story than with the product. Ultimately, we are storytellers.'

As someone who strongly believes in the restorative power of coffee, Jonathan doesn't have to convert me, nor explain any further intricacies of his business. We have known each other for a long time and we share similar passions. But when I think about Bean There coffee from now on, it will be about Agnes and her story.

'I met Agnes in Kenya,' Jonathan told me. 'When I sat down with her for the first time, we chatted and we connected well. A little while into the conversation, I went down the line of "How many kids do you have? Tell me about your life", which is a general direction a conversation often takes. I discovered that she had two kids, a son and a daughter. At the time, Anne, her daughter, was still in school but her son was not in school. She said that the reason he was not in school was that she did not have the bucks. She had to choose who could go to school. At that point, my natural reaction might have been the reaction of most people having connected so well with someone, namely, to say "What can I do to help you out?" Then take out my wallet and ask how much school fees cost. But I found myself thinking back that the reason why I am here is to trade fairly with Agnes. Fair trade is about trading and not about charity. We started to buy Agnes's coffee and we have worked with them for about twelve years. We paid fantastic prices, not because it was charity or anything, but because it was deserved. Their coffee is the finest on the planet. Agnes at that time was getting involved in agronomy training, getting good farming practice training. Because she was so motivated, she got equipped and properly stuck into the training. She ended up increasing her own yields in coffee. She became so involved in the agronomy training that she started training her neighbours. She became a promoter farmer. She started going around and showing people how to look after their trees. She got recognised in her community as a leader. As a result, in the last two or three years, she became district chief in her community.'

Jonathan then fast-tracked to a recent visit to Agnes in Kenya.

'When I first met her she had a small mud hut. This time we sat in a brick home with a tin roof and gutters, electricity, appliances, nice furniture. She cooked us an amazing meal. She came and sat next to me and said, "I want to show you the history of our relationship," and she pulled out from her Facebook profile pictures of us back in 2007. Scrolling through and seeing that process and the visits, I thought, wow. We stepped outside and the local vet was there inseminating one of her cows. Agnes had no cows before. I just stood back and thought, look at that progress.'

Jonathan's smile at the end of the story said it all. 'That is the story I use to tell about fair trade,' he said. 'Obviously, that is not the story for everyone. We have disasters and we have successes. But people remember that story about Agnes and what fair trade is about. They ask me, "Is this Agnes's coffee?"'

Lauren Moss, in her narrative therapy work, has seen extraordinary breakthroughs in some of her clients through how story can shift thinking and allow them to construct a new narrative for their lives going forward. 'One of the things I do in the first session, I ask them what their goals are for the therapy process. I write them down and we leave them. Then we do the story and we engage in the therapeutic process. Then I start looking out for words they use. I also write in the session, I literally write what they are saying and as soon as I start seeing words change, then I will start reflecting this back to the client. Instead of saying, "Let us change your story from victim to survivor" – because there is a part of the brain that goes "No, we need the victim's story. We need to heal in that. We need to define ourselves in that" – rather than being directive, I wait. People are amazing because they will pop those words out.

'I remember one client. She never called her rape the rape. She would just say "the incident". One day she said it. The rape. It was so powerful because suddenly it had a name and we could put it on the shelf somewhere. She would be like "Yes, this thing happened to me." It was a thing. So in those moments, I reflect back and say, "Have you noticed that you called it something different? Have you noticed that you have started to talk about yourself differently? You are starting to use words like "I deserve".'

Lauren feels therapy should be 'a gentle process'. 'Usually when someone comes to therapy,' she explained, 'there has been harm and injury. To be able to look at that, you are already changing your story.'

In my interview for this book with Ivan Moroke we talked about the story of our country and the importance of understanding and acknowledging the past and present narratives of the nation's people. I shared with him some of my feelings about 1994 – some dreams shattered and some dreams that came to pass. I asked him how he believed our story as a country might unfold and he gave me his view.

'The apartheid legacy is going to be with us for a while,' he said. 'It was a brilliant architecture, if we can call it brilliant in terms of making sure the legacy continues. It seems like since the new dispensation, the country is more divided than it has ever been. This has not just happened. If you consider the euphoria of the Mandela era, we have to ask ourselves – so what are the real reasons that we flipped? Race relations are much worse than in 1994. Much worse. So what is it? It did not happen by mistake. Either there is something we did or something we did not do. Something was done that got us to where we are.

'Maybe the new story that should be told should be about dealing with and being far more directed to 1994. Maybe let us talk about our storytelling from people's realities since 1994. If we are trying to find solutions about "Why are we where we are?", maybe that is a story that happened and that is a different 1994. The story, I suspect, will be different for different people. What has been the story since then in terms of their expectations and fears and how things have turned out? There is a need to get to grips with this period of our story in order to craft a new story going forward.'

Ivan's words resonate with what Anele Nzimande said to me with regard to a new generation: 'We need to be transcending pain versus defining ourselves based on pain and trauma.' Ivan believes the new story can be combined with the old – 'so that there is context of where we came from'.

Referring to the 'What's Your Story?' programme, he said: 'I think that is what I like about what we are doing. The storytelling is always followed by specific things – tangible things that an organisation has to do. That is the single biggest thing about the storytelling because without that, it is just a once-off feel-good talk shop. It is the follow-up action that is needed. If you think about it, it reflects what happened to the country. The emotional part during the Mandela era; the techno-craft part during the Mbeki era. It has a natural progression. To do the emotional and understanding is one thing, but what is the key thing now?'

Ivan used the analogy of a research organisation such as Kantar, the company he heads in South Africa, and the client. 'Giving the client the facts and the data of where they are, that is important data, but you become a partner if you can tell them that with this data, here is what you can do to effect growth in the company.'

'Ultimately, research is about understanding the story,' I said.

Ivan responded, 'That is exactly it. It is about understanding who, where, how, why. Why do people do what they do? So that companies can make decisions and strategies and plans. They can defend the threats or explore the opportunities. It is the "Now what?"'

'The client is looking for the story of the past and the present in order to craft a future,' I said. 'You cannot craft a future by ignoring the past.'

'Exactly,' said Ivan.

EPILOGUE

It's a beautiful, jasmine-infused spring afternoon. It's my favourite time of year, when the exuberant colours of jacaranda and bougainvillea compete to wash out Johannesburg's winter brown. A time for new beginnings.

I've left work early to have tea with my mother. She doesn't know it, but this is no ordinary visit. We've spent the last few years encouraging people to get to know each other's stories in order to debunk our assumptions and judgements and build understanding. Then I'd had this early morning revelation. What about me? How much did I know about my own parents' story? Precious little, was the answer. Ironically, was I not guilty of having judged them without knowing their story? Dad had recently died so that chance had gone but Mum was still alive.

I arrive at her home, my home for so many years, prepared to ask.

Mum is sitting on an antique sofa in her living room. In fact, everything in the room is antique, Mum included. She's just turned 82.

I look at this woman, my mother, with the sunlight streaming through the window creating a halo around her newly permed hair. I can't remember a time when Mum's hair wasn't permed. In fact, I have no idea whether it was originally straight or curly … it's brown now; I think that might be her original colour. She is still an attractive woman. Great genes, English mist and expensive cosmetics have bequeathed on her a smooth skin that makes her look much younger than her years.

I battle with my emotions towards her, as my love and admiration contest with anger and dislike.

'Darling,' Mum says in her plummy voice, borrowed from the Queen, 'you want to interview me? About what?'

'About your life, Mum,' I say gently.

She looks at me down her aquiline nose. 'Mmm …' she muses, 'not sure there's much to tell … Met your father, moved to South Africa … had you children and now here I am.' There is finality in her voice.

This wasn't going to be easy, but I already knew that. Mum is a product of her generation. One does not talk about oneself, especially not to one's children.

'Oh, come on, Mum, there's clearly more,' I say.

'Well, what else do you want to know?' she asks, slightly irritated.

I tell her I want to know her story. Things like her childhood in England, about her parents, her marriage to Dad, and more about me growing up.

A glimmer of a smile crosses her face. She knows she's cornered. 'Oh, all right then,' she relents. 'When do you want to start?'

'Now,' I say, sitting down beside her.

Sixty years ago, my mother was the English girl who captured my South African father's heart. After serving as an officer in the Second World War, Dad went to Oxford to read Law. It was on a skiing holiday with friends that he first spied the young woman who would become his wife. She was standing with a group in the hotel they were all staying in.

'Is that girl in the green jersey with your party?' he asked her tall aristocratic cousin. 'Because I would like to invite her to come out dancing with us.'

Having had a year at school in England, I had experienced first-hand how the English upper classes believe themselves to be innately superior to anyone who is not English, landed, titled or born in the Home Counties. They wore them easily, their prejudices, against anyone not like them – against Jews, Catholics and, in particular, people of colour. Was it this arrogance that had enabled them to rule over a quarter of the world?

In any event that was Mum's heritage. I would so have loved to have watched as this slight, olive-skinned, bespectacled caricature of a Jewish man, my father, made his preposterous request. Mum's cousin wanted Dad to get lost, little knowing that this would play straight into Mum's rebellious streak. So, 'the girl in the green jersey' went dancing that night.

'What were your first impressions of Dad?' I realise I am curious to know my mother's answer.

'Well, he didn't speak English,' Mum says.

'What do you mean?' I ask, puzzled.

'Well, not proper English. He spoke with an accent!'

We both laugh a little, imagining, before Mum continues. 'But he was so different to the other young men one met then. I just couldn't imagine being married to any one of the chinless wonders that used to frequent our set. And then your father came along and …. well, you know!'

'Did anything happen that holiday?' I ask playfully.

'Happen? What do you mean happen?'

'Oh, come on, Mum,' I say, exasperated.

'Well … there was some stoodling … in the corners.'

'Stoodling?'

'Yes … you know,' Mum says with a sly smile, the colour rising coyly up her cheeks.

I am 46 years old and somehow the concept of my parents 'stoodling' makes me feel uncomfortable. But then again, I did ask.

After that holiday Mum went back to London. Six months later she married my dad.

'That was quick. What did your family think?' I ask her.

'They were horrified,' she says. 'After all, he was Jewish! My father sat me down and didn't quite say he would disown me, but he made it clear that your father was not like us and that would only bring me trouble. I suppose he was right, because as soon as our engagement was announced in *The Times*, I received four hateful anonymous letters accusing me of betraying my class.'

This was 1949, just four years after the end of the Second World War. Wasn't the Holocaust still fresh in people's memories? Did they have no shame?

Mum seems unmoved as she recounts the story. I can't help wondering why. I would have been spitting mad if I had been treated like that. But she has this weird dissonance. She seems sympathetic to the letter writers as, being anti-Semitic herself, she might also have been outraged if one of her 'set' had married a Jew. I've lost count of the number of times I've pointed out the irony of her anti-Semitism and marrying a Jew. Each time I was met with her stock reply: 'But that's different!' until eventually I gave up. Prejudice defies logic.

'And your mum, what did she think of Dad?' I ask.

'Oh, she was just so relieved that I wasn't marrying a Catholic,' she says.

You've got to be joking, I think to myself, but she's not. I decide to move on. 'And Dad's family?' I ask.

Mum ponders a while and then she says, 'Well, your grandfather was disappointed that I didn't have any money.' Then she adds, with vehemence, 'Nasty little man.'

Mum can be accused of having many faults, but being duplicitous is not one of them. If she doesn't like someone, that is that and they know it. In this case, I think her judgement was correct. My grandfather was, from all accounts, a 'nasty little man'. Witty, intelligent, a great raconteur and a great divorce lawyer. So good that he comforted three of his clients by marrying them. His fifth wife was ten years younger than him. By all accounts he was a distant and uninvolved father who, after divorcing my grandmother when Dad was six, left the parenting of my father and his sister to their governess.

The light has turned golden, signalling in some unwritten way the time for tea. Mum leans over to pour it. As she grips the tea-pot I am reminded of her age. Her hand that was once smooth and full is now translucent and sagging, the anatomy clearly visible.

'So, Mum, I'm going to tell you what I know and you're going to fill in the gaps. That okay?' She nods.

'You were born in 1923 to two artists,' I begin.

'Yes,' she says. 'Mummy and Daddy were both studying art in Paris. Not sure how or why they got together, but it was a very "free" time, when people were throwing off the shackles of conventions and trying out all sorts of things.'

'Including relationships?'

'Probably,' she says. 'Soon after they met, they married, and shortly after that they had me. Jolly silly of them. Neither of them were at all suited to being married or being parents, so their marriage didn't last.' I nod. This much I knew.

Mum was sent to live with her grandmother. She was looked after by a nanny for a while and then shipped off to boarding school.

She was five years old.

I am incredulous. Boarding school at age five? I dropped out of nursery school at five ... I still had cot-sides ... I am trying to imagine it – such a little girl going off to boarding school, alone.

'And your parents?' I ask softly. 'How much did you see them?'

'Not much,' Mum replies. 'I used to see them about once a year, usually at Christmas.'

When I ask her what happened during the rest of the year, a faraway look comes over her face. 'That was a bit hard ... I remember waiting at the school gate on the last day of term. I was never sure who was going to come and pick me up ... It was usually my cousins. I spent most of my holidays with them.'

As she is speaking, my heart beats faster. I'm feeling the fear of that little girl, suitcase in hand, alone at the school gate, wondering whether anyone is coming for her. I'm beginning to understand her a little more and some of the anxiety that has rubbed off on me.

We ramble onwards, with me asking, probing, listening. Her childhood was not awful, but with all the moving of places and relationships there would have been nothing to make her feel anchored or secure in who she was. Maybe that was why she so thoroughly embraced being English upper class with its mannerisms, accent and prejudices. To give herself an identity and a narrative she could belong to.

'I need a short loo break,' Mum says, breaking into my thoughts. I watch her manoeuvre herself off the sofa. It is always a performance; first she positions her stick to assist her good leg, then she finds a handhold and finally, with her good arm, heaves herself up.

'Can we talk about your polio when you get back?' I ask, and she shrugs in acknowledgement as she limps away.

As a child, one of my earliest memories was of listening to Mum's step, thump, step, thump as she walked down the passage to say goodnight to me. Then, when I was older, of holding my hand behind my back so that she could steady herself as she walked. I had never known her as able, but always as uncomplainingly disabled.

Mum reappears and repeats the performance in reverse: stick positioned, handhold and then let go as she collapses back onto the sofa. We begin again.

'You'd been in South Africa for about five years when you contracted polio?'

'Thereabouts, yes,' Mum says. 'I developed a high temperature and went to our GP and he prodded and poked, as you doctors do' – she gives me a meaningful look – 'and then he said, "Well, you could at least turn yellow!" before sending me home. I think he wanted a nice sign like jaundice so that he could label me' – another meaningful glance. 'The next morning I couldn't move my legs. Daddy phoned our GP, who said it was in all likelihood polio. And so I was rushed straight off to the fever hospital. The paralysis spread to my right arm and to the left side of my face.'

Although she is recounting this quite dispassionately, my imagination fills in the gaps. 'It must have been incredibly scary,' I say.

'Yes, it was a bit,' says Mum. 'Ghastly place. Doctors would come and talk about me as if I wasn't there. "Get the iron lung ready, she'll soon need help breathing." "Such a shame, two small children and unlikely to walk again." And so they continued.'

I know the hospital. Wards with long, cold, brick-clad walls, rows

222

of iron beds with their accompanying beige lockers made of tin. How frightening it must have been for her. Apart from her husband, she was alone in a foreign land. She had yet to make friends.

'They said I would either be in a wheelchair or would always need two sticks.' Mum continues matter-of-factly. 'And they also said that it would be dangerous for me to have any more children.'

They weren't wrong about the last part. She would have been much more susceptible to complications in pregnancy and childbirth. But my mother had always wanted a big family and she was undeterred by the physicians' dire predictions. Soon she was pregnant with my brother. What were she and Dad thinking, I can't help wondering. But whatever issues I may have with my mother, I also can't help but admire her immense courage and bloody-mindedness.

We are interrupted by Leonora bustling into the room, her work uniform swishing around her generous figure. She is a cheerful woman in her mid-40s. She is here to collect the tea-tray and bring a blanket for Mum to insulate her from the late afternoon chill. For the last three years, Leonora Ngwenya has cared for Mum as if she were her own mother, so continuing a line of women who have been in our family's lives. Serena Mojapelo was for me the most significant of them, because it was she who was the constant warm presence in my formative years. My memories of my own mother are patchy in those years, probably as a consequence of how our brains are wired, linked more to traumatic events and hard times. I take this opportunity to ask Mum about some of these times.

'Mum, why, when I was at junior school, did you refuse to let the school barber cut my hair?' I ask, still remembering the humiliation of being the only boy in the school who had a note from his mother on haircut day.

'Well, you had such beautiful hair, darling,' Mum says serenely. 'I didn't want some barber to destroy it.' For the second time this afternoon I am incredulous.

'I was a boy, Mum, not a shrub! Did you ever think what the impact on me was to be the only boy whose mummy wouldn't allow him to have a haircut?'

From her silence, I think the answer is no. I'm also angry that Dad never challenged her. I'm on a roll, remembering ... 'And did you ever think about the impact that your anxiety for my safety would have on me? Your constant refrain of "Don't get hurt", "Be careful, that's dangerous" were like a dripping tap that made me constantly fearful.'

Silence. Uncomfortable, Mum adjusts her blanket to break the tension of the moment and then she says, 'I'm sorry you felt that way.'

It's the best I'm going to get from her.

I have a flash of insight. The separation anxiety that had dogged and shaped me in my formative years, was rooted in *her* fear, not mine. Her fear of losing me. My mother was, in essence, an abandoned child. The vision I had of her on the last day of term, unsure who, if anyone, would be there for her, is still strong. Maybe that experience fuelled her subconscious need never to be abandoned again. Was it this that had led to her unhealthy attachment to me? But why me and not my siblings? I'm not sure I'll ever know the answer to this, if there is one. I may still be angry at Mum for her selfishness but I am beginning to understand where it came from.

I wish I'd asked my father why he let Mum be so over-protective, but he died a few years back, so I will never know why he didn't intervene. You always think there will be time to get your parent's story from them and then it's too late. My parents had a complex relationship. I'm not sure how happy they were, but with both of them having come from broken homes, they had decided never to leave each other, no matter how bad things might be. I am grateful to them.

The afternoon is drawing in. I move onto safer ground.

'Russia, Mum. Tell me about learning Russian and your trip to Russia at the height of the Cold War. I remember coming home from school in the 70s after another day of being fed a steady diet of the "rooi gevaar"—'

'The what?' Mum stops me mid-sentence. I forgot that despite having lived in South Africa for over 50 years, she pretends not to understand a word of Afrikaans.

'"Red danger"', I translate. 'Fear of communism. I came home from school one day with all this ringing in my ears to find you studying Russian and preparing for a visit to Moscow. Are you sure you weren't a spy?'

The tension of the preceding minutes is broken and we both laugh. 'I just found the language, art and literature fascinating,' says my mother, who barely finished school.

We continue to talk about her Russian trip, how despite pushback from some of her friends, who had wondered about her true motives, she had, unafraid, gone alone.

I can see that she is tiring and I suggest we carry on another time.

She pulls a face. 'Not sure there's more to tell,' she says.

'That's what you said when we began two hours ago,' I say with a smile. 'I think we're just getting started.'

I get up, it's getting dark, and I draw the curtains. Mum reaches for her embroidery. I turn on the overhead lights and the lamp next to her. At the door I turn and look back. My mother is already bent over her work and she doesn't look up. At a glance, what would you see? A small crumpled figure in a pool of light, a woman, old now and nearing the end of her life. Mother. It's an ordinary word and everybody has one. But wrapped inside that ordinary word is so much more. This woman is the source of so many conflicting emotions in my life. Through the example of her life, she taught me so much about courage and perseverance, and she introduced me to faith. But, at the same time, her infectious anxiety and her deep need to keep me close had a devastating impact on me.

The time we have spent together this afternoon has quite fundamentally shifted things for me. I will not understand it fully right away, but with the dawning of greater understanding has come an acceptance. It is very easy to blame Mum. However, if she'd thought about it, she would have blamed her mum, and her mum would have blamed hers and so on. And none of them would have felt any better. So forgiveness is not only the right thing, it's the sensible thing.

Now I feel more sad than angry, sad for us both, I suppose. She mothered me the best way she knew how. In many ways, I know how fortunate I have been to have had her in my life.

'I love you, Mum,' I say from the doorway.

She looks up and smiles. 'Love you too, my boy.'

REFERENCES AND SOURCE MATERIAL

Campbell, Joseph. *The Hero with a Thousand Faces*. New York: Pantheon Books, 1949.

Cole, Ernest. *House of Bondage*. New York: Random House, 1967.

Friends in Recovery (edited by Kathleen W.). *Twelve Steps to Freedom: A Recovery Workbook*. California: Crossing Press, 1991.

Denning, Steve. 'The Science of Storytelling'. *Forbes* magazine, 3 September 2012.

Gottschall, Jonathan. *The Storytelling Animal: How Stories Make Us Human*. Boston: Mariner Books, 2013.

Heminway, John. *In Full Flight: A Story of Africa and Atonement*. New York: Alfred A. Knopf, 2018.

Ho, Ufrieda. *Paper Sons and Daughters: Growing up Chinese in South Africa*. Johannesburg: Pan Macmillan, 2011.

Kirsten, Deborah. *Chai Tea & Ginger Beer: My Unexpected Journey … Cricket, Family and Beyond*. Cape Town: Struik Christian Books, 2015.

Lewis, CS. The Chronicles of Narnia (series).

Lewis, CS. *The Lion, the Witch and the Wardrobe* (The Chronicles of Narnia, Book 2). London: Harper Collins, 1993.

Paton, Alan. *Cry, the Beloved Country*. Vintage, 2002.

Sacks, Jonathan. *Morality: Restoring the Common Good in Divided Times*. BBC Radio 4 Podcast, 2018.

Tolkien, JRR. *The Lord of the Rings*. London: Allen & Unwin, 1954.

White, Paul. Jungle Doctor series.

Woods, Donald. *Biko*. London: Paddington Press, 1978.

CONTRIBUTORS

Michael Charton qualified in South Africa as a chartered accountant and spent time in a financial consulting role in the United States. His passion for history led him to read extensively and then to discover the art and power of storytelling. He saw storytelling as a channel through which to make South African history more accessible to a broad range of audiences. He is the founder of Inherit South Africa, an enterprise that aims to reveal important, untold stories from South Africa's past for entertainment and nation building. He developed and performs the show *My Father's Coat*, using story to take a fresh look into South Africa's past.

David Dennis, a graduate of UCT Drama School, is an actor who has won a significant number of awards for classical, contemporary and musical theatre across the almost four decades of his career. One of his most notable, long-running roles was as Sol in Soul City. He is currently head of the Live Performance School at AFDA Johannesburg.

Laura Dison has worked at Wits University as a teaching and learning specialist for 28 years. In 2020 she was appointed Assistant Dean, Teaching and Learning, in the Faculty of Humanities and co-ordinates the post-graduate diploma in Higher Education, which is a professional teaching qualification for Wits lecturers. In 2010 she helped establish the Wits School of Education Writing Centre and has worked with Education lecturers to design embedded writing interventions in disciplines to enhance students' reading and writing practices.

Buhle Dlamini is a sought-after international consultant and facilitator in the fields of the future of work, diversity and organisational culture. As an entrepreneur he was named one of the Future100 Entrepreneurs in South Africa. He is co-founder of numerous non-profits, including Columba Leadership SA, Heartlines and forgood.co.za. He holds a certificate in Fundamentals of Strategy from Harvard University and is a fellow of the Cultural Intelligence Center in Michigan. He is the author of six books, the most recent being *Unleashing Your Greatness*.

Lillian Dube is a multiple award-winning actor, with two Lifetime Achievement awards, from Duku Duku as well as Naledi Theatre awards. She played the part of Sister Bettina in Soul City for over ten years. In 2017 she received the highest national honour in Lesotho and in 2018 she was given the National Order of Ikhamanga.

Khayelihle Dom Gumede is an award-winning actor and director for theatre and television, who is a BA (Dramatic Arts) graduate from Wits University. In 2012 he was a recipient of a GIPCA Emerging Theatre Directors Bursary, and was honoured with a Naledi Theatre Award in 2015 for Best Director for his interpretation of *Crepuscule*, the dramatisation of a Can Themba short story. He was co-director of *Tsotsi, the Musical* in 2018, which was based on the eponymous Athol Fugard novel. Currently he is the chief operating officer of Clive Morris Productions and the chief creative officer of Yililiza.

Alison Harris is an art director and design thinking consultant based in Cape Town. With a strong background in ad agency art direction, she founded Sk8 for Gr8 in 2014, a social enterprise aiming to build creative critical thinking in children through skateboarding. She is the creative director at children's book publisher Imagnary House.

Ufrieda Ho is a journalist who reports and writes for a number of publications and titles on a broad range of issues. She is the author of *Paper Sons and Daughters*, an acclaimed memoir on growing up Chinese in South Africa, which she wrote at a time when the country was awaiting its democratic dawn.

Deborah Kirsten graduated cum laude from UCT with a Bachelor in Primary Education and a Master's degree in Theory and Philosophy of Education. She has worked as a freelance journalist for a number of publications, and is the author of the book *Chai Tea & Ginger Beer*. Along with colleague Jacqui Mol, she developed and teaches a course and workshop entitled Living Your Strongest Story and, more recently, Growing Your Strongest Story, a workshop designed specifically for teenage girls.

Brent Lindeque is the founder of the online Good News site and he is the Good Things Guy. He was a LeadSA Hero, was selected as one of Africa's Most Promising Entrepreneurs, and was one of the prestigious *Mail & Guardian* Top 200 Young South Africans. His creation of three dedicated feeding schemes in Canada, the United States and Ireland are still running to this day.

Zolani Mahola is a singer, actor, inspiration speaker and agent for social change. She was a founder member of the pan-African, multi-cultural, multi-genre band Freshlyground in 2002, one of Africa's most acclaimed and successful bands. The band opened stages for and collaborated with artists such as Stevie Wonder, BB King, Hugh Masekela, Miriam Makeba, Robbie Williams, Oliver Mtukudzi, Vusi Mahlasela and Busi Mhlongo. Zolani has expanded her portfolio to include what she terms Inspiration Talks, in which she shares intimately about her life story and the challenges she has faced.

Olefile Masangane is a worshipper, husband, father, motivator, facilitator and a passionate communicator. He works with Heartlines as a programme manager, mobilising churches and institutions in South Africa to move from professed values into lived values. He holds a BA in Communication Science from UNISA, is a certified mBIT coach, and a Cultural Intelligence facilitator with the Cultural Intelligence Center in Michigan in the United States. He has contributed to youth development through organisations such as Youth for Christ, the Salvation Army, Young & Able and Columba Leadership. He has also consulted with Adopt-a-School Foundation in facilitating strategic planning and team-building processes for schools.

Gcina Mhlophe is an author, poet, playwright, director, performer and storyteller, who has performed all over the world in theatres such as the Royal Albert Hall and the Kennedy Centre. Her collaboration with Ladysmith Black Mambazo and the Francis Bebey quartet, Africa at the Opera, toured opera houses in Germany. Her autobiographical play *Have You Seen Zandile?* earned her the Fringe First Award at the Edinburgh Festival, the Sony Award for Radio Drama from BBC Africa, and the Joseph Jefferson Award in Chicago. She is the founder and director of the Zanendaba storytelling company. She has received honorary doctorates from the London Open University, the University of KwaZulu–Natal, the University of Pretoria and the University of Fort Hare. She is currently the executive director of Gcinamasiko Arts & Heritage Trust. Gcina's birthday – on 24 October – has been recognised as National Storytelling Day and is celebrated all over South Africa.

Ivan Moroke is the CEO of Kantar Insights Division, South Africa, part of Kantar, the world's leading data, insights and consulting company. He has held leadership roles at global advertising agencies Lowe Bull and TBWA Hunt Lascaris, and was group managing director at Yellowwood Future Architects. He was the founder of the marketing insights and strategic consultancy, Co-Currency. He is the ex-chairperson of the jury for the APEX Awards, ex-chairperson of Brand Council South Africa (BCSA) and ex-vice-chairperson of the Association for Communication and

Advertising (ACA). He sits on judging panels of other industry awards, the Loeries, Bookmarks and Marketing Achievement Awards. He sits on the boards of the Nelson Mandela Children's Hospital Trust and Kantar South Africa. He is chairperson of Heartlines.

Lauren Moss is a counselling psychologist with professional experience in the NGO, academic, tertiary education, corporate and private practice settings. Her primary focus is on treating adults and couples in her private practice.

Steven Mzee is a pastor at Every Nation Church in Cape Town. His passion is to see God's people live out their God-given talents and giftings. Born and bred in Kenya, he graduated from the Mombasa Polytechnic University and obtained the Certified Public Secretary Certification; he also has certificates from the His People Bible School and Every Nation Leadership Institute.

Seth Naicker is managing director at indi-Afrique training and development, an associate of Heartlines, part-time faculty at the Gordon Institute of Business Science, and ordained into pastoral ministry. He is a dynamic facilitator and inspired communicator, whose specialty is reconciliation and inclusivity in the workplace. He has a Master's degree in organisational leadership, and applies his practical and academic learning in his professional consulting and coaching career. Seth, his life partner Merrishia Singh-Naicker and their children go about their family life in faith, hope and love. Together they have served in South Africa and abroad with a key focus on healing, transformation, justice and reconciliation.

Anele Nzimande is a law graduate of Wits University. In 2016 she joined the Centre for Applied Legal Studies as a legal researcher in the Business and Human Rights unit. She is a published author, content creator and communications specialist.

Quinton Pretorius is a speaker, trainer and team-building facilitator who lives and breathes diversity. As a youth leader in the 90s, he travelled to schools, reformatories and juvenile centres, discovering the depths of division and imbalance between different segments of society. He served on the international Youth for Christ team, Ithemba, and became the deputy director of the programme. He was the co-ordinator of the Siyithemba Project, which sought to transform schools and equip students and teachers to achieve academic excellence; he has been a fellow of the Clinton Democracy Fellowship Programme, and has had an association with both the Gordon Institute for Business Science (GIBS) and Heartlines.

Irene Robinson was born in Denmark and emigrated to Canada with her family at the age of three. She came to faith in Christ at the age of 18 and later studied at Prairie Bible College in Alberta, Canada. She and her husband Leigh have served in pastoral ministry in South Africa and Canada for over 40 years, with a focus on building community in their churches using their gifts of hospitality and networking.

Jonathan Robinson began his working career in the IT industry with IBM and Dimension Data. In 2002 he joined the Starfish Foundation and followed his desire to impact the future generations of South Africa by helping to create a brighter future for orphaned and vulnerable children. In 2005 he combined his passion for Africa with his love for coffee and established the Bean There Coffee Company. Bean There is South Africa's first roaster of certified fair trade coffee and works with small-scale farmers in Ethiopia, Tanzania, Rwanda, Burundi, Kenya and the DRC.

Leigh Robinson was born in Johannesburg, and committed his life to Christ in Sunday school at the age of nine. He studied at Prairie Bible College in Alberta, Canada. He and his wife Irene have served in pastoral ministry in South Africa and Canada for over 40 years.

Jonathan Shapiro (Zapiro) is one of South Africa's best-known cartoonists. He has been published in the *Mail & Guardian, The Sowetan,* the *Sunday Times,* Independent Newspapers and the *Times,* and is currently editorial cartoonist for the *Daily Maverick.* He has published 25 best-selling annuals and four special collections, and has won numerous international and South African awards for his work. In 2019 he was appointed Chevalier de l'Ordre des Arts et des Lettres (Knight of the Order of Arts and Letters) by the president of the French Republic.

Jimmy Volmink is Dean of the Faculty of Medicine and Health Sciences and professor in the Department of Global Health at Stellenbosch University. He has previously served as the founding director of Cochrane South Africa, as well as the founding director of Research and Analysis at the Global Health Council in Washington, DC. He received a Harvard/ South Africa Fellowship, obtained an MPH from Harvard University, and was subsequently awarded an Oxford Nuffield Medical Fellowship to study at Oxford University, where he obtained a DPhil degree in Epidemiology. He is widely recognised for his contributions to evidence-based medicine. He is an elected member of the Academy of Science of South Africa and an elected Fellow of the Royal College of Physicians of Edinburgh. He has also received the Leverhulme Medal from the Liverpool School of Tropical Medicine and a Recognition Award for his contributions to evidence-based health care in Africa from the South African Medical Research Council.

ACKNOWLEDGEMENTS

I have always loved reading beautifully written books but I have never appreciated what gifting and skill goes into their writing, until now. Unsurprisingly, in measuring my efforts against theirs, I often wanted to pack this in. That I didn't is due to the many people who have walked this journey with me and encouraged me when I flagged. They say it takes a village to raise a child; well, in my case it took an assortment of very special people to write this book. I want to thank them for their faith and encouragement, which enabled this book to see the light of day.

In particular, I want to thank Andrea Nattrass and Terry Morris from Pan Macmillan for not only believing that this book was worth publishing but for engaging Alison Lowry to assist me. They must have known that it would need a person like Alison, with skill, empathy and perseverance, to shape the book, find a way to incorporate the material in the interviews I conducted, and shepherd it into being.

Thanks to my Heartlines colleagues and board for their encouragement and support and for seeing this book as an extension of our work to encourage people to share their personal stories. In particular, Derek Muller, Zamabongo Mojalefa, Brian Helsby, Thabisa Dyala, Olefile Masangane, Latasha Slavin, Pamela Kgare and Nevelia Moloi for encouragement and feedback; and Jennifer Charlton, who read everything and gave me great feedback, including, 'Garth, this chapter is boring!' And she was right!

To my friends who got me through medical school: Denis Turner, Megan Cole, Cheryl Attree, Mike Wilkinson, Eric Baasch, Guy Date and Tracy Jamieson.

Behind every man who thinks he is successful is a woman who really is. My wife Jayne, the unsung hero of my story, who encouraged, cajoled and gave me insightful guidance, reassurance and the time to write.

My children Rebecca and Leigh have been wonderfully supportive and mildly surprised when their dad's response to, 'So when are you going to finish the book?' changed from 'Well, uh, I'm not that sure …' to 'It's finished!'

To my sisters Dee Tobin and Xanthe Williams for believing that their 'little brother's' book should see the light of day. To my brother Miles and sister-in-law Jetje. Their support over many years has made much of my story possible.

To my colleagues at Soul City from whom I have learned so much, Sue Goldstein and Shereen Usdin. Their generosity of spirit also allowed me to take sabbaticals to explore ideas.

To Harriet Perlman, Janet Berger, Kathi Walther Bouma, Camilla Leeds, Susan Bentley and Gisele Crewdson for taking the time to read drafts.

To Michael Cassidy, Graeme Codrington, Ufrieda Ho, Gcina Mhlophe, Lillian Dube, Gary and Deborah Kirsten, Jonathan Shapiro and Michael Mol who kindly reviewed the book.

A real highlight in writing this book was the opportunity to interview a range of diverse and extraordinary people who gave generously of their time and shared their stories about story with me. My only disappointment is that I was not able to use more of their stories as their interviews alone make for compelling reading. So thank you Alison Harris, Anele Nzimande, Brent Lindeque, Buhle Dlamini, David Dennis, Debbie Kirsten, Ufrieda Ho, Gcina Mhlophe, Ivan Moroke, Jonathan Robinson, Jonathan Shapiro, Khayelihle Dominique Gumede, Laura Dison, Lillian Dube, Olefile Masangane, Professor Jimmy Volmink, Quinton Pretorius, Steven Mzee, Zolani Mahola, Lauren Moss, Leigh and Irene Robinson, Michael Charton and Seth Naicker.

Many thanks to Debbie Wright for helping set up and manage the interviews and to Dimakatso Songoane for transcribing the many hours of transcripts.